AN INTRODUCTION TO

Trans/DSD Athletes

Anthony J. Catanese, MD FACS

Published by Wheatmark®
2030 East Speedway Boulevard, Suite 106
Tucson, Arizona 85719 USA
www.wheatmark.com

ISBN: 979-8-88747-169-3 (paperback)
ISBN: 979-8-88747-170-9 (ebook)
LCN: 2023924029

ordering discounts are available through Wheatmark,
or more information, email orders@wheatmark.com or
888-934-0888.

This book is not a substitute for medical care or treatment. Medicine should only be practiced by a licensed, trained professional. Opinions expressed here are that of the author and are based on his experience. They do not reflect the view of any organizations—medical, sports, political, or otherwise.

The subject of trans athletes is in a state of rapid social change both positively and negatively. It is essential that any subject in this book be checked against current socio-political and medical knowledge. If factual information is required on a subject, it should be obtained from the original document.

At this point in time, there are few high-quality studies about trans/DSD individuals. This is particularly true of studies involving testosterone and its effects on athletic performance. Most of the information in this book is based on the author's experience and common medical knowledge. The lack of references is one weakness in a text on this subject.

To all the trans and DSD athletes
who have endured ignorance and rejection
throughout their journey.
Keep persevering!

Contents

Preface

This book contains information that should be common knowledge for urologists or sports medicine physicians. Medical terms are explained as they are used so that the book remains friendly to nonmedical readers. It is meant to be an educational work to spark discussion. Specific references are avoided. Material included is from information the author used in forty years of practice.

When the author lectures on and explains the concepts discussed in this work, the reaction is always the same. The audience members admit they were poorly informed prior to the lecture. Many of the attendees are then willing to view the subject differently and have an open mind.

Acknowledgments

Editors	Elaine Wallace, Alfonso Moreno, Wilfred Chabier
Contributors	Neel Shah, MD; Nick Patel, MD; Josua Sterling, MD; Adam Kane, APN
Artwork	Catherine DeLeon

1

The Trans Athlete

Introduction

The reader may want to skip to chapter 2 and read definitions before starting the book.

In the United States, 0.6% of adults are trans, approximately 1.6 million people. The number is greater among high school students and is estimated to be up to 5% when including nonbinary students—those with neither a male nor female gender identity.

This is a controversial subject, and it is essential that the reader keep an open mind before rushing to any conclusions or making any judgments. A true understanding of the issue requires the reader to abandon the concept of two sexes that cannot be changed and replace it with a concept of multiple sexes that are fluid and mutable.

When a trans person is accepted and supported, they thrive and are successful. When they are rejected, they suffer significant psychological stress. While the solution in sports may not be as simple as people on different sides of the argument think, it is still necessary to treat trans people with respect and dignity.

The author's main medical practice is as a urologist. Urologists, and more specifically pediatric urologists, are the surgeons who treat differences (disorders) of sexual development (DSDs). Plastic and reconstructive urologists are the surgeons who perform sex-confirmation surgery. While I do not perform that surgery, one of my partners is a large-volume sex-confirmation surgeon in the New York area.

The information in this book is current and medically sound. The challenging part of caring for trans individuals involves navigating the social and political issues they are up against. This is true in various countries, including the United States. The purpose of writing this book on trans athletes is to educate people and to start a conversation.

The subject of trans athletes and the rules governing their participation in sports are in a constant state of change. In recent years, there have been multiple rulings made internationally by organizations such as the International Olympic Committee (IOC), nationally by Congress, and locally by state governments. There are also individual sports organization rules. These rules are often contradictory, inconsistent, and until recently, not sport-specific. They will be discussed in more detail in upcoming sections. DSDs and gender dysphoria are included in the same book because their treatment and many of the implications overlap. It is not that the two are the same thing. DSDs are medical disorders, with some confusion as to the gender of the child, in which abnormal levels of hormones naturally occur and may be necessary for the health of the individual. Gender dysphoria occurs when there is a volitional desire to have one's physical appearance changed to best match the sex they identify with—simply put, to change their sex. It is often associated with voluntary changes in hormone levels. Both trans and DSD individuals are likely to encounter obstacles in sports because of birth sex, gender identity, and hormone levels.

The following discussion may be more detailed than most nonmedical people require, but since there is so little literature and information on this topic in the sports-medicine community, it is important to establish a reference for future policy.

I wrote this book because I became disgusted with the treatment of my trans and DSD patients. The mistreatment has been mostly sociopolitical and not medical. Medical treatment is solid as long as there are no barriers to its availability. In 40 years of practice, I have had several trans patients, including teenagers, who died by suicide. Current thought now is that over 50% of gender-dysphoric teenagers have contemplated suicide. This is because they feel helpless and abandoned by the system.

Anybody who denies the existence of transgender individuals might feel differently if they had a better understanding of the subject. More about this is discussed later in the book. I am certain that with knowledge, one can develop a deeper understanding of the issues and become more open-minded toward transgender people.

The existence of people with DSDs is often easier to digest because it is a congenital medical problem (i.e., one that exists at birth) that, if not treated, can result in serious medical consequences and possibly death. It is not by choice and not psychological, but these individuals often have gender dysphoria and often require the same hormonal and surgical interventions that trans individuals do. The experience of treating people with DSD has caused many healthcare providers to accept trans people. Physicians who treat trans people generally believe it is a medical condition. Since gender dysphoria is a medical diagnosis, its treatment can be covered by insurance.

Trans athletes are another, more complicated issue. There are many physicians who believe in and treat trans individuals but do not support trans athletes. Only with knowledge and debate will the issues surrounding trans athletes come to a resolution.

Philosophy of Caring for Gender Dysphoria

When I started medical school, I had never heard of a trans person. Going to medical school in New York City, I was quickly introduced to the variety of different people in the world. I treated patients with different ethnicities and races as well as social and political views. I was exposed to patients with medical and psychiatric conditions and physical disorders. Often the medical problem was self-inflicted from alcohol or drug use. There were healthcare providers who were not comfortable taking care of these patients who were different than themselves. These physicians had to quickly accept the notion that the job was not to judge but to care for all patients. If they could not make this transition, they often dropped out of clinical medicine and went into a field without patient contact. Given the number of trans people in the United States, it is impossible for a physician to not come in contact with them. It is the duty of the physician to care for the trans patient just like they would any patient. If the healthcare provider rejects trans patients, they should not be practicing clinical medicine.

2

Definitions

I was taught that a definitions section in a book is redundant and unnecessary because the book itself will explain the definitions. However, this subject is unfamiliar to most readers that a section on definitions is probably welcomed.

How to Address a Trans Person

Trans people are addressed with the honorifics (*Mr., Miss, Mrs.*) and pronouns (*he, she*) consistent with their gender identity. The only caveat is that a nonbinary person is sometimes addressed as *they*. Ask if you do not know, and try not to act surprised. Progressive medical institutions have all the pertinent questions on their patient registration form. The healthcare providers should read the forms and ask the patient if it is unclear. In some states, the patient's legal sex may be different than their chosen trans designation. This is because some states in the United States and some medical insurance companies will not recognize a transgender identity until legal paperwork has been completed.

There may be certain waiting periods for legal change. Most states are currently allowing the change of sex on a birth certificate with some simple paperwork.

Trans Terminology

These definitions are listed in an order that is helpful when reading the book.

Genotype—This refers to someone's genetic makeup. While it is used to refer to sex chromosomes in trans literature, it includes all chromosomes and associated genes. For our purposes, it is biologic sex with XX being female and XY being male.

Karyotype—This refers to an actual photograph of a set of someone's chromosomes. This is sometimes used interchangeably with *genotype*.

Phenotype—This refers to observable and physical characteristics of a person and their appearance. If someone appears to be male, they are phenotypically male. If someone appears to be female, they are phenotypically female. This includes the appearance of their secondary sex characteristics and sex organs. XX appears as a girl/woman and XY as a boy/man. The genotypic sex and phenotypic sex usually match, but that is not always the case. When there is a mismatch between the genotypic and phenotypic sexes or when the phenotypic sex is unclear, the child is said to have ambiguous genitalia. This is the case with DSDs. In the past, this was also termed *intersex* or *pseudohermaphrodite*. *Intersex* means "between the sexes," and *pseudohermaphrodite* means "appearing to be both sexes." Both of these terms are no longer preferred. One's phenotype is based on one's appearance and has nothing to do with the genotype.

Gender/Gender Identity—This is the sex that a person feels and thinks they are. It can have little to do with the phenotypic and genotypic sex, although in most cases, the three of them are the same. Most people identify with one or the other of two sexes, but that is not always the case.

Nonbinary—This is an increasingly common gender identity whereby the individual identifies as a gender that cannot be exclusively identified as male or female. This does not come up too often in sports but serves to illustrate how complex the subject can be.

Gender Expression (Presentation)—This is how an individual expresses their gender identity through appearance, dress, and behavior.

Gender Dysphoria—A mismatch between someone's birth sex and gender identity with the associated distress.

Gender Confirmation—This is discussed in more detail further in the book. It can be understood as the confirmation of gender identity and expression. Besides appearance, dress, and behavior, it is accomplished with hormone administration and gender-confirming surgeries.

Gender Nonconforming—A person whose behavior or appearance does not conform with the prevailing cultural and social expectations about what is appropriate to that gender. It may also be called *gender fluid, gender queer,* or *gender diverse.*

Detransition (Desistance)—To change gender identity back to the birth-assigned gender identity.

Sexual Orientation—This refers to the sex that someone is attracted to regardless of their genotypic or phenotypic sex. If one's gender identity is male and he is attracted exclusively to women, he is heterosexual. If his gender identity is male and he is attracted to men, he is homosexual or gay. If her gender identity is female and she is attracted to men, she is heterosexual. If her gender identity is female and she is attracted to women, she is lesbian, homosexual, or gay. If a person is attracted to both men and women, they are bisexual. It is said that sexual identity is who you go to bed as, and sexual orientation is who you go to bed with. Although this expression has been criticized for being crude, it explains the situation very well.

Orientation Summary—The frame of reference is based on one's gender identity.

    Heterosexual—Attracted to the opposite sex.

    Homosexual—Attracted to the same sex.

Gay—Male and sometimes female homosexual person.

Lesbian—Homosexual woman.

Bisexual—Attracted to both males and females.

Asexual—Attracted to neither.

Pansexual—Gender-blind, attracted to all sexes; a more universal orientation than bisexual.

Questioning—Unsure if other than heterosexual.

Queer—Refers to all alternative sexual orientations and gender identities.

Straight—Heterosexual.

LGBTQ+—Lesbian, gay, bisexual, trans, queer, and more. The reason the T is included in the acronym is because the initials are inclusive of all alternative genders and orientations.

Differences (Disorders) of Sexual Development / DSDs—This occurs when a person's genotypic sex does not match their physical appearance or their genitals. In the past, these individuals were called *pseudohermaphrodites* or *hermaphrodites* or *intersex*. In modern discussion, *hermaphrodite* is not used when discussing humans; although *intersex* is more acceptable, it still feels uncomfortable for the DSD patient who identifies strongly as male or female and should not be used. Both of these terms have been replaced with the term *DSD*. This originally stood for *disorders of sexual development,* but *differences of sexual development* is preferred by many with such conditions.

Many DSDs are genetically based and will be discussed later in their own chapter. People with DSDs include individuals genetically one sex, genetically a combination of two sexes, or genetically missing some aspect of a sex. They can appear as one sex or the other. They can be XX, XY, or have three or more chromosomes. They can be missing an X chromosome (XO). Many of these people have hormones, whether naturally occurring or artificially induced, that are in conflict with the sex they appear to be.

In the past, these individuals were raised as whatever sex they most looked like, the default sex being female because it is easier to remove genitalia and create a vagina than to construct a penis. There were horror stories about children being raised as one sex and later on identifying as another. Today, this is not what is done; instead, a child with a severe disorder is allowed to grow up and establish their own identity. They are raised as the sex they feel most comfortable as, with gender-confirmation surgery being performed at a later date. A child's gender identity is usually solidified by the age of six but can be formed as early as two.

Transgender Surgery (Sex-Change Surgery)—Both terms exist in medical literature and are considered archaic and problematic. Trans people do not change their sex but alter their bodies to conform with their gender. A trans person is a trans person regardless of whether they can change their body presentation or not. In medical discussions, *sex-change* and *transgender surgery* have referred to the change of one's physical appearance through the use of surgery and hormones. The correct terms are *gender-confirmation surgery* and *gender-appropriate hormone replacement,* but one needs to be aware of the older terminology in order to read the literature.

Trans Persons—*Trans male* describes someone who was assigned female at birth whose gender identity is male, whereas *trans female* describes someone assigned male at birth and whose gender identity is female. A *cis male* is someone who was assigned male at birth and whose gender identity is male, and a *cis female* is someone who was assigned female at birth and whose gender identity is female. Sometimes the terms *trans person, trans boy,* and *trans girl* are used. *Nonbinary* is gender identity that is neither completely male nor female.

When trans issues were originally discussed in sports medicine, most people thought that one's sex was determined by their DNA and their biological organs. There were no exceptions to this. In other words, whatever sex you were genetically, that is the sex you were. Later on, the community started to consider different points of view and believed that an individual who physically changed their gender presentation through surgery and sufficiently changed their hormone levels through artificial means could be counted as the sex that aligned with their identity. The change in belief was based on a deeper understanding of political, social, and human rights issues.

Subsequent to this, it was realized that there were limitations on an individual's ability to alter their primary and secondary sex characteristics because of cost, difficulty in achieving the desired surgical results, and availability of treatment in different parts of the world. The position then was the individual's gender presentation needed to be consistent with their gender identity, and they needed to achieve hormone levels consistent with the average levels for the gender for a certain period of time. Legal sex change and surgery were not necessary as long as gender identity was achieved.

Sex Characteristics—*Primary sex characteristics* are one's genital appearance. *Secondary sex characteristics* are hip and breast development in a female and muscle, deepened voice, and a beard in a male. Secondary is caused by hormones and primary by genetic makeup along with hormones.

Gender-Confirmation Surgery—This was formerly known as a *sex-change operation,* which is considered an archaic, inappropriate term. Gender-confirmation surgery is performed on individuals with DSDs to convert medical problems associated with these disorders and on individuals with gender dysphoria. The DSD patient will often undergo surgery and hormonal treatment as a child. This surgery may be medically necessary because the associated conditions can be life threatening. Sometimes the gonads, testes, and ovaries in DSD patients can form tumors. Gender-confirmation procedures often follow since the known gender identity is established by the age of six.

In gender dysphoria, gender-confirmation surgery is often delayed until the individual is of legal age to make the decision. This is usually 18 in most states but is sometimes younger. Puberty-delaying drugs are often included for children as long as they are legally available where they reside. More about this is discussed later in the book.

For trans individuals, the process of transitioning involves three parts: social transitioning, which means presenting themselves to society in a manner congruent with their gender identity; hormone transitioning, which means exogenous hormone supplementation; and surgical transitioning, which involves surgery to achieve phenotypic sexual characteristics.

DSD patients whose anatomy may include a combination of male and female sex organs or incomplete development of certain sex organs often require gender-confirmation surgery to confirm a gender identity. It may also be necessary for medical reasons as some of the DSDs can lead to cancer formation if certain parts of the anatomy are not removed. They may also medically require medications or hormones to survive.

The reason people with gender dysphoria and people with DSDs are often grouped into the same medical categories is because there is a great deal of overlap in terms of treatment, which may seem to be the same thing to a nonmedical individual.

Barr Body—The Barr body was discovered in the 1960s, and the Barr body test was the first test used to determine an individual's genotypic or chromosomal sex. The test detects an inactivated X chromosome. A female individual has two X chromosomes (XX), and a male individual has an XY pattern. Because a girl/woman has two X chromosomes and only requires one, the extra X chromosome is often deactivated in the individual. This is not the case for the other 44 chromosomes, for which two copies are usually needed. The inactivated chromosome can be detected with special staining as a clump of DNA in the person's blood. A stain is a coloring agent put on a piece of tissue to be viewed under the microscope. It is a relatively easy test to perform. The presence of the Barr body identifies the individual as a genotypic female.

The test first became available in the 1960s—state-of-the-art technology at the time—and scandals immediately arose because some Eastern European / Soviet bloc female athletes tested negative for Barr bodies, which meant they were genetically male. Females are positive for Barr bodies because they have an extra, inactivated X chromosome. Remember, females are XX, and males are XY. Males are negative for Barr bodies because they have one functional X chromosome as well as a Y chromosome. This is mostly of historic interest as newer tests are used now, but it illustrates how determining someone's genetic sex has become a simple procedure only in recent years.

Crossdresser—Someone who desires to wear clothing associated with the opposite sex sometimes for erotic reasons, usually heterosexual. It has nothing to do with trans people.

Transvestite—Archaic term for *crossdresser*.

Drag Queen—Theatrical performance often for charity, sometimes for political agenda, where a gay person dresses as an exaggerated persona of the female sex. This has nothing to do with trans people.

Testosterone or Androgens (Male Hormones)—Testosterone is at the center of the trans/DSD athlete debate. If it were not for the issues with testosterone levels in athletes, particularly those who identify as female with levels of testosterone above the normal range, there would not be much controversy.

Testosterone is a naturally occurring androgen, or male hormone. Cis women have a much lower level of testosterone than cis men. Women's testosterone is produced by their adrenal glands and ovaries. Levels are listed later in the text.

Exogenous supplementation of testosterone has traditionally been prohibited by the World Antidoping Association (WADA). Recently, the acceptance of DSD and trans athletes has allowed testosterone supplementation within certain limits. WADA has also initially tolerated abnormal levels in female DSD athletes because it was a naturally occurring phenomena. This is no longer the case. Limits on testosterone levels in DSD athletes have recently been established. It must be emphasized that there is a paucity of studies on testosterone, and most of the above statements are extrapolated from other sources.

Testosterone has many effects physically and possibly on psychological development, particularly when it is present during puberty. Males are generally 15% larger than females. This includes muscles and bones that result in greater strength but also involves the heart and lungs because the heart is a muscle and the lungs require muscles such as a diaphragm to function. There is also evidence that testosterone can result in more aggressive behavior as well as body size and muscular development, which may not revert back to pre-testosterone levels after the testosterone is removed. The saying is that "testosterone is forever." This is why there is such interest in postponing or blocking puberty in trans adolescents.

These changes are of concern in power sports, but there is evidence that they are also relevant in endurance sports such as long-distance running. This is because testosterone increases the red blood cell count and levels of hemoglobin in the cells. Hemoglobin is the red pigment in the blood that carries oxygen. The higher the testosterone, the higher the level of hemoglobin. This is the reason testosterone is abused by endurance as well as power athletes. When oxygen delivery is improved in these athletes, so is their performance.

Attempts to divide up sports like distance in track to those that are more testosterone dependent and independent are flawed. Many people believe that all sports can benefit from testosterone. Indeed, psychological behavior is strongly based on testosterone.

Also of concern is the trans male who never had testosterone present at puberty. He will never become as strong as the cis male who had it present. Attempts to play catch-up with testosterone do not have the same effect after one is done growing. There is also concern regarding small amounts of fetal testicular testosterone in utero—in other words, while the baby is developing. This is in addition to mini puberty. Mini puberty is a larger concern and will be discussed in future sections. The simple presence of a Y chromosome may also be a factor.

All of the above are reasons this is of concern in contact sports. There is the danger of the cis male injuring the trans male or the trans female injuring the cis female. This has led sports physicians to believe that some sports may be acceptable for trans athletes and some not. Sports have been mandated by the IOC to make their own individual DSD/trans policies. The IOC realizes all sports are different and that they must make their policy.

Drugs Used in the Treatment of Trans/ DSD People

Most of the drugs discussed in this section, with the exception of estrogens, are on the WADA prohibited list.

If an athlete was prescribed one or more of these drugs, they would require a therapeutic use exemption (TUE) for each of them. A TUE will often be granted as long as the drug was prescribed in the therapeutic (normal) range. This is particularly true of a drug like testosterone in the trans male. Determining what the minimal ranges of testosterone are for different groups is the challenging part.

The individual sports organizations, along with the United States Antidoping Association (USADA), would be the ones to report the TUE. WADA becomes involved with international competition.

Aromatase Inhibitors—In the human body, testosterone is broken down to estrogens by an enzyme called aromatase. When someone is administered testosterone, there is a rise in estrogens from its breakdown. This is an unwanted side effect. It can result in things like gynecomastia, or breast swelling. Many trans men are on an aromatase inhibitor along with testosterone.

Cortisone—This is a large group of drugs both natural and synthetic. They are naturally produced by the adrenal gland. In adrenal cortical hyperplasia (ACH/adrenal genital syndrome), there is a genetic defect where one of the enzymes in the adrenal gland is defective or absent. This can be a life-threatening situation. The problem can be corrected with the administration of cortisone or an additional similar drug. It may be a lifelong administration and require a TUE. These patients may also require a mineral corticoid, which is a drug that helps the body retain salt. A TUE, of course, is required.

Cyproterone Acetate—This is an oral (by mouth) drug used to block pituitary hormones, which tell the testes to make testosterone or the ovaries to make estrogen. It has many uses in medicine, but it is not usually used in the United States because of its side effects. Lupron has replaced this drug because it is safer and more reliable. The advantage of cyproterone acetate over Lupron is that it is cheaper and oral. Lupron is expensive and parenteral (by injection).

Estrogens—These are prescribed to trans women. While there is no monitoring of estrogen levels, it is important that they be given an appropriate dose because the side effects of the administration can be serious and may induce blood clots. Estrogens and related drugs usually do not require a TUE because they are the main component of birth control pills, which are not on the WADA prohibited list. Nevertheless, many sports medicine physicians recommend a TUE anyway. Most trans men, if they have not had a hysterectomy, need to lower their estrogen levels with Lupron. Estrogens may be given as a pill, shot, patch, or cream.

Lupron (Leuprolide Acetate)—Lupron, along with half a dozen other formulations of the same or similar drugs, is an injectable anti-puberty drug administered every one to six months depending on the formulation. Lupron is actually a brand name, but it is universally used to describe this group of drugs, so it will be used throughout this book. This was originally developed as a prostate cancer drug to lower testosterone, which is the fuel for prostate cancer. It works to stimulate the pituitary to stop making luteinizing hormone, which is sent from the pituitary to the testes or the ovaries and results in the cessation of testosterone and estrogens, respectively. It functionally puts a stop to puberty and is best administered as soon as a child has been psychologically designated as trans. Starting the drug in adulthood or after puberty would be helpful and necessary before the administration of trans hormones, but results are best if puberty can be avoided. This way, there is no development of secondary sex characteristics, which make transitioning a more difficult process.

Criticisms of the drug include its cost (approximately $125 a month) and potential side effects. Side effects include a small chance that puberty will not resume when the Lupron is stopped. It should be noted that the detransition rate for trans children is only a few percent, so this is an uncommon concern.

Other side effects include osteoporosis and possible increase of bone fractures and also slightly taller stature. This is because testosterone has broken down estrogens, and estrogens are responsible for the fusion of bone and growth plates. Without estrogens (testosterone), bones are thinner and longer. People treated with Lupron for puberty delay tend to be taller but not out of place.

In fact, Lupron is used to delay puberty in congenitally short-statured children in order to get them to grow a few inches taller. It is also used in children who are developing into puberty too fast. This will help them achieve normal height. Health insurance generally pays for Lupron in this case and the pediatric endocrinologist who administers the drug. This is often the same physician who treats trans children.

Anti-trans advocates feel Lupron is too serious a drug to be given to children. It can be used to prevent puberty until the child is of legal age to obtain surgery. This is usually 18 years of age or can be younger in some states.

It is worth discussing Lupron and its effects on prostate cancer. Prostate cancer requires testosterone for growth. In the 1940s, it was discovered that if someone with metastatic (spread) prostate cancer was castrated (removed testicles), the prostate cancer would regress (shrink) for usually about two years. Lupron today is used instead of castration. Someone on Lupron has a testosterone level of under 40 mg/dL. Since the average age of the patient with prostate cancer is 66, a patient usually has a baseline testosterone of about 250 mg/dL. If one lowers the testosterone level to 40 mg/dL in 66-year-olds, some of them have very few side effects, but many have side effects. The side effects are very variable, but most have an obvious loss of muscle mass and increase in body fat. This is sometimes so severe that it will put a man into heart failure because the heart is a muscle. Athletes in particularly seem to have more severe symptoms including loss of strength and severe fatigue. Every urologist who treats prostate cancer knows this and tries to use the drug sparingly. There is evidence of a strong role of testosterone in strength and muscle development as demonstrated here. It should be noted that the serious side effects usually only occur in those who are elderly and rarely in a trans adolescent.

Mineral Corticoids—This is a large class of drugs that are sometimes needed in ACH (adrenal cortical hyperplasia) patients in addition to cortisone. They prevent the loss of salt in the urine, which could be life threatening. They require a TUE. There are many different formulations, and no specific names are mentioned.

Progesterone—Another female hormone produced by the ovaries. It is often a component of birth control pills. Birth control pills usually do not require a TUE, but this drug is sometimes used along with estrogens in trans women, and a TUE would be required.

Proscar—Also called *finasteride*, it is used in both trans males and trans females to prevent hair loss. It inhibits the enzyme 5-alpha reductase and will be discussed in detail in the section on DSDs. Given before puberty, it can cause a decreased development of male sex organs. If it is given postpuberty, it prevents the development of baldness and prostate growth. It is never given to reproductive-age women because of its side effects on the male fetus. It may not currently be on WADA's antidoping list, but a TUE is advised anyway.

Spironolactone—This is actually a diuretic, which is a drug that causes urine loss. Its anti-testosterone effects were described as a side effect. As a diuretic, it is often avoided in young males for that reason. It is sometimes used to prevent hair loss in cis women. It blocks the conversion of testosterone to 5-hydroxy testosterone, which is the active form, for secondary sex characteristics in cis males. This is an enzyme that is missing in the DSD 5-ARD.

It is often used in the initial treatment of trans women. It is inexpensive, oral, and available worldwide. It may also be used in combination with other drugs in polycystic ovary syndrome (PCOS). It is excellent at preventing testosterone-induced hair loss. In countries outside the United States, it is administered with cyproterone acetate instead of Lupron. In the United States, it is often given with Lupron. It requires a TUE because it is a diuretic and can be used to disguise other illicit drug use.

Testosterone—This is the principal androgen in the human male. It is primarily produced by the testes. The adrenal glands in both men and women, along with the ovaries in females, make a small amount of testosterone and other androgens. Most of these androgens are not as potent as testosterone.

Testosterone is the only legal androgen for which a TUE can be obtained. It is the center of the trans athlete controversy. Its effects are potent and not completely reversible if stopped. This is a potentially abusable drug, and its prescription requires close monitoring. The appropriate levels in both trans and DSD athletes, both male and female, are uncertain and are constantly changing. The high potential of abusability of testosterone is a validation for its performance effect. This will be discussed more in future chapters.

3

Introduction to Genetics

Basic Genetics

When I took genetics in college, James Watson and Francis Crick had only just discovered DNA 25 years earlier. I actually had no formal genetics classes in medical school.

The plans for building the human body are contained in the chromosomes, which are composed of DNA. The DNA is translated into proteins by the body during development and during repair and rebuilding. Some proteins are structural like muscle and bones, and some proteins are enzymes. Enzymes make processes in the body happen. An example would be testosterone causing an increase in muscle growth. A muscle itself is a structural protein, and the testosterone is an enzyme—more specifically, a hormone.

There are 46 chromosomes, two sets of 23, one set from each parent; 44 are called autosomes, and two are called sex chromosomes with XX being female and XY being male. Together, they are known as the genotype. A picture of the chromosomes is called a karyotype, which is a term sometimes used interchangeably with *genotype*. It is the Y chromosome that determines maleness.

DNA is a complex subject, and attempts to simplify it often miss important information. Here, we are trying to keep the subject simple and relevant to trans/DSD athletes.

The reason genetics is so important is because most DSDs have a mutation, a defective or an absent gene (DNA instructions). This results in an absent or defective protein or enzyme. It can also be a defective group of genes. We have identified many, although not all, of the DSD mutations. No specific genes for gender identity have been identified, but we know a percentage of people behave as if they have a genetic or inherited basis. This can be inferred by population and twin studies. More of this will be discussed later.

The body has two sets of chromosomes and therefore two sets of genes (DNA instructions). The DNA is ultimately transformed into proteins. This involves RNA and protein synthesis, which we are going to skip for now. All we need to know is that chromosomal DNA and genes are the plans for making protein in the body. Each chromosome contains a massive amount of DNA. Its genes are instructions. While we have been able to map out the entire human DNA, we still do not understand what a lot of it does or how it works.

Recall that we get one copy of the gene from each parent. Some genes are so strong that one copy can dominate over another, and some are weaker, but both copies are needed. An error or a mutation in the gene might have no effect, or it may have a profound effect. It depends on the gene. The body is so complex that an altered gene that produces an altered protein could be fatal or could have no effect.

Because chromosomes carry massive amounts of DNA, the loss of a chromosome or even a small part can have profound developmental effects and is often fatal. The one exception is the X and Y chromosomes. When a female child is born, they have an extra X chromosome because they get one from each parent, but mostly only one is needed. The extra plays a small role, but it is not fatal if absent. The Barr body, which was discussed earlier in the definitions, is the extra inactivated X chromosome that can be found in the blood and is an indication of XX, which is the female genetic sex.

If an individual is missing an X chromosome but has one from the other parent, the individual is XO or has Turner syndrome. YO is nonviable (not able to live) because too much information is contained in the X chromosome to survive without one. If someone has an extra X chromosome, XXY, they have Klinefelter syndrome and also have some abnormalities, but they are viable. Both Turner and Klinefelter syndromes can be classified as chromosomal DSDs but rarely come up in the discussion of trans/DSD athletes. I have described them here as an illustration of the complexity of genetics. There are other sex chromosome abnormalities, but they are very rare, and many are fatal.

Mosaics are a mixture of chromosomes. It is a little complex to understand but worth knowing. Normally, every cell in the body has the same chromosome. In a mosaic, parts of the cell—say, 20%, 30%, or 40%—have one set of chromosomes, and the remainder has a different set. There are many ways this can happen, and we will get into that. An example would be 46 XX/XY, which is a mixture of female and male. This is a true hermaphrodite (both sexes). In the animal kingdom and in humans, it is more appropriately known as ovotestis syndrome. The child has sex organs of both sexes. While rare, this is the ultimate DSD. These patients often require corrective surgery to remove the gonads because of the high incidence of tumor formation.

In the past, these children were surgically made into the female sex because it is easier to remove tissue than to add it on. Their genetics are most often in a mixed state, not really both sexes. The subsequent gender identity assignment results were mixed, and in some studies, they were only as good as a coin toss. Today, these children are allowed to choose their own identity, which they do by two to six years of age. There are very little detransitioning and few gender-identity issues if this plan is followed.

When a gene is said to be "sexed linked," it means it is on the sex chromosome, X or Y, and not on the autosomes. DSDs occur "sexed linked" as well as autosomal dominant and recessive. The genes involve hormone receptors, hormone levels, hormone function, and often the appearance of the external genitalia.

Genetic Abnormalities

It is good to go over genetic abnormalities again because it can be such a confusing topic. The chromosomes are made up of DNA, which makes up the genes and is the plan for protein synthesis. The protein is the structure, hormone, enzymes, and chemicals that make up and maintain the body. Most genetic abnormalities are not due to chromosomal abnormalities but due to gene abnormalities. Many of these abnormalities have not yet been identified. The abnormality can be a missing gene, a defective gene, an extra gene, or a seemingly unrelated gene and even on a different chromosome that modifies the gene's function. This can result in too little of, too much of, or the wrong protein, which is often a hormone for our purposes. Since there are two of each chromosome, one from each parent, there are two genes or two sets of instructions for the protein. There are several scenarios of how these genes may function. They may both function, one may function over another, they may both be defective, or one may produce a good protein and one a bad protein. This can result in normal, partly abnormal, or completely abnormal proteins. The gene function can be influenced by another or sometimes distant and seemingly unrelated gene. This gene can be on the same or a different chromosome. It can be very complex, and we are just starting to understand how it works.

Y Chromosomes

The Y chromosome is responsible for maleness. In the absence of the Y chromosome, the individual is female—XX being a normal genotypic and usually a phenotypic female and XO being a Turner syndrome female with some incomplete development. Turner syndrome produces a number of congenital anomalies, and people with it are usually short in stature and infertile. XXY, or Klinefelter syndrome, is another viable chromosomal abnormality, and the individual is male because of the Y chromosome.

The Y chromosome contains instructions for male genitals, including the testes, which produce testosterone. The Y chromosome also contains the directions for some male traits that are testosterone-independent. The full extent of the DNA information on the Y chromosome is not completely understood. An example of this would be stature or height. Male infants tend to be 15% larger than female; although testosterone is present in utero and during mini puberty, some of the height difference is thought to be independent of the testosterone.

There is not a large amount of genetic information on the Y chromosome when compared with the X chromosome or the autosomes. The Y chromosome has about 80–200 genes, whereas the X chromosome has about 900–1,400 genes. The Y chromosome is not necessary for viability (life), but it is for maleness. One X chromosome is required to be viable. Besides male genitals (testes), testosterone, and stature, there are other, less well-understood traits on the

Y chromosome. For example, the Y chromosome codes for hair on the ears and exclusive male traits.

Y chromosome sexists have suggested that the male has something that the female does not. The rebuttal is that it is possible to live without a Y chromosome but not without an X chromosome. Remember that a human being needs one X chromosome to be viable but not a Y.

The Advantages of a Y Chromosome

There are many advantages of the Y chromosome. Some are mediated through testosterone, and some are independent. There is controversy over which effects of the Y chromosome are mediated independently of testosterone. Testosterone has an effect in utero and particularly during mini puberty. It has a profound effect in adolescent puberty and throughout life. Many of the effects are in part permanent.

Males are larger than females and have more muscle strength, including endurance, more pulmonary (lung) capacity, and more cardiac (heart) capacity. They have longer bones, which result in more leverage and, subsequently, strength. The differences are estimated to be about 15%.

The most interesting differences involve neurological development. Some of this development is thought to be hormonal or testosterone dependent, and some of it is due to the Y chromosome. Critics of testosterone explain different behaviors involving parent expectations and social upbringing. It is the nature-versus-nurture argument. Males are generally more aggressive, which is an advantage in sports. Whatever the cause, this is an issue that must be relevant in the evaluation of the trans athlete. In the schoolyard, boys get into more fights than girls, even prepuberty. In the United States, males commit murder at a rate seven times greater than females.

When trans men compete with cis men, there is a concern that the cis male can injure the trans male because of these factors. These include physical as well as mental injuries. This is particularly true in contact and weight sports.

The Y chromosome has a sex-determining region (SRY) gene, which is a code for the testes. The testes make testosterone. The testosterone has the effects discussed above in utero, mini puberty, adolescent puberty, and throughout life. The Y chromosome also has effects by itself such as size and possibly other less understood issues, independent of testosterone.

Mini Puberty

Another concern in our development is what is termed *mini puberty*. During gestation (pregnancy), a small amount of the mother's pituitary hormones, which are medically necessary to maintain the pregnancy, cross the placenta and allow the infant's gonads (ovaries or testes) to make small amounts of sex hormones. This goes on throughout pregnancy but particularly in the third trimester. The fetus actually makes estrogen and testosterone. The hormones cause development of the infant's secondary sex characteristics in addition to other facts that we have limited knowledge of, such as neurologic development.

It is not unusual to have some breast development and

even menstruation in female infants. Males can have genital development, pubic hair, and even erections. Other effects of these hormones are mostly unknown. In the male, there is increased bone, muscle, heart, and lung development. Most of these secondary sex characteristics regress in three to six months, but some effects of the testosterone are believed to be permanent.

There are DSDs called androgen insensitivity syndrome (AIS) and 5-ARD, the first of which lacks functional testosterone receptors, and the second of which is defective in the levels of functional testosterone. There is a variable that often limits the effect of mini puberty. The effect of the Y chromosome is still present and unknown. A complete AIS might have very little mini puberty, but each athlete needs to be evaluated on an individual basis. The effects of mini puberty in the DSD 5-ARD are unknown.

One of the controversies in the trans athlete debate is the effect mini puberty has on the physical and psychological development of the male infant. Girls have little or no testosterone. They have estrogen and progesterone along with growth hormone, and the pituitary works in a similar fashion, although it is not believed to be as potent as testosterone.

One of the debates involves testosterone's effect on neuropsychological development, particularly aggressive behavior, which appears to be a benefit in all sports. Proponents of this, despite the example of prepuberty male children getting into more schoolyard fights beyond the level that would be accounted for by social norms, also note that prepubertal males tend to be more aggressive in contact sports. There is a large surge of interest in contact sports at the time of puberty, even in trans athletes who have had natural puberty blocked. There is thus some concern over mini puberty and its psychological effects.

Six Levels of Maleness

The following are six levels of maleness that can be addressed by opponents of trans female / DSD athletes. Some can be altered or prevented, but some cannot.

1. Presence of Y chromosome
2. In utero testosterone
3. Mini puberty
4. Adolescent puberty
5. Long-term effects of puberty
6. Psychological effects of being raised male

In the trans female, there is no way to alter numbers 1, 2, and 3, although 4, 5, and possibly 6 can be prevented. DSD athletes have a variable group of disorders, and while they may have a Y chromosome, 2, 3, 4, 5, and 6 are all variable. The main concern is the presence of male puberty and the persistence of testosterone.

4

Testosterone

Measurement of Testosterone

Testosterone levels are the main concern when discussing trans athletes. Testosterone is measured differently in other parts of the world, and this makes the literature very confusing. In the United States, testosterone is measured in nanograms per deciliter (ng/dL). In Great Britain, Europe, and most of the rest of the world, it is measured in nanomoles per liter (nmol/L). The way to convert one to the other is by dividing the world measurement by 0.0347 or multiplying the US measurement by 0.0347.

This is very technical, but it is essential to anyone trying to interpret the literature on testosterone. In the United States, an adult cis male's testosterone level is between 250 ng/dL and 1,200 ng/dL. This number can vary slightly depending on which lab is used. It is highest at puberty and declines through the male's life. Unlike estrogen during menopause in women, testosterone does not reach a very low number. Replacement of testosterone in aging men is generally not mainstream medicine. A cis woman's testosterone level is between 15 and 70 ng/dL, although this number is not well understood. A small amount of testosterone is made by the female adrenal glands and ovaries.

The following is an example. A testosterone level of 10 nmol/L in Europe, which was the acceptable DSD level until 2022, divided by 0.0347 would be 288 ng/dL, which is the lower natural male level. This number was not obtained by any scientific study but by political consensus. It seems that the number is at the low end of the male range. Recently, this number has been changed to 5 nmol/L, which is 144 ng/dL in the United States. Both of these numbers are still very high for an average woman. Recall that the normal number would be 15–70 ng/dL for a cis woman. While 5 nmol/L is more reasonable than 10 nmol/L, it is still high. Testosterone is known to have effects at very low levels. Most recently, some organizations have required a DSD athlete to have a level of 2.5 nmol/L. This would be 72 ng/dL, a very reasonable level and compatible with cis females.

Later in the book, we will discuss PCOS, a disorder that is sometimes classified as a DSD that is not uncommon in female power athletes. Rarely does an athlete with a PCOS have a testosterone level much higher than about 100–140 ng/dL.

Other Hormones

Testosterone, the male hormone, is produced primarily by the testes. It is also produced by the adrenal glands and the ovaries and is present in small amounts in the female.

Testosterone is a hormone that is part of a large group of hormones called androgens. Sometimes the words *testosterone* and *androgens* are used interchangeably. There is at least one other form of testosterone naturally occurring in the body, dihydroxy testosterone. Dihydroxy testosterone is a more potent form of testosterone that is responsible for secondary sex characteristics such as facial hair and genital development. Most of this is discussed in the DSD section under 5-ARD.

In addition to testosterone, there are other growth hormones. There is estrogen from the ovaries in females and a very important growth hormone called human growth hormone (HGH), which is produced by the pituitary gland. It has a strong effect on the development of strength in concert with estrogens and testosterone. Women's ability to grow muscle strength is a combination of HGH, estrogens, and adrenal androgens along with numerous other growth factors that are made throughout the body. This is sometimes an argument used against the importance of testosterone, but it is flawed because if a woman is given testosterone, she will become stronger than women without testosterone supplementation. It is important to remember that there are many hormones and growth factors in both sexes that work in concert, some of which are well understood and some of which are not. Testosterone is a major factor in strength and endurance.

Facts about Testosterone

Testosterone functions in a large range of blood levels. It is very high around the time of puberty and drops as a man ages. The level in a 65-year-old can be 20% of the level in puberty, and this is still considered normal. Some of the effects of testosterone include the lifelong maintenance of male secondary sex characteristics and function. There is also a surge effect at puberty and young adulthood. There is some evidence that men become less aggressive as they age and their testosterone levels decrease. It is well established that adult strength and endurance decrease with age. It is estimated that adult strength decreases at a rate of 10% per decade starting after the third decade of life.

Attempts to supplement testosterone in older adult athletes is of limited value because athletic performance depends on multiple factors. This is not an argument against the value of testosterone in athletic performance; it is just a caution. Supplementation of testosterone to above physiological levels in young to middle-aged men can definitely improve some parameters of strength and endurance. In trained athletes, it can definitely improve performance. It must be remembered that the supplementation of testosterone in cis males as well as cis females is a violation of WADA's antidoping rules.

Bodybuilders often abuse androgens, both testosterone, which they take in massive doses, and other androgens and sometimes veterinary formulations that are very strong. Surprisingly, most bodybuilding competitions are not drug-free. While it is difficult to compare a bodybuilder with other athletes, there are some similarities. The athlete tries for strength, power, and performance; the bodybuilder primarily for hypertrophy definition and fat loss. While bodybuilders are strong, be it for a different goal than other athletes, it is clear they can develop subsequent size, strength, and decreased body fat. How they stack up against other athletes is very variable. It must be remembered that all sports are different, and one thing that is clear is that testosterone causes muscle growth.

In the trans male, testosterone supplementation is appropriate within the range of the cis male. People on testosterone have an increase in medical conditions including blood clots and increased red blood cell count. Sometimes it is necessary to periodically remove some blood and/or place the patient on a blood thinner such as aspirin. It is important to realize that the increased blood count and associated hemoglobin, which carries oxygen, improve endurance, which is one of the major reasons endurance athletes also abuse testosterone.

Testosterone traditionally has not been available in the United States as an oral medicine but as an injection, patch, or gel. It was also expensive. Recently, a new oral formulation of testosterone has become available in the United States. Oral preparations have always been available outside the United States, but there were concerns about side effects including liver disease, and they were limited in the United States.

When an athlete's performance is evaluated, it is found that trans females are still performing at an above average level when compared with cis females two years after the reduction of their testosterone level. This is why it is felt that some of the testosterone effects are permanent. This stresses how important adolescent puberty is in the trans athlete debate. Despite this, until recently, many organizations only required two years of testosterone reduction in the trans female athlete.

The level of testosterone necessary to achieve in order to participate as a trans female athlete is constantly changing. One surprising constant is that, while it needs to be lower than in cis males, it often does not need to be as low as a cis female. This is in part because the reliable way to reduce testosterone to this low level is castration (removal of testicles) or administration of Lupron. Castration is permanent, and Lupron is expensive. Neither of these options is available to everyone, particularly in other parts of the world. It is important to remember that anatomy and hormones are not required for gender identity. It is instead presentation and feeling of body image with the desired sex—in other words, how comfortable one is with oneself.

The required hormone levels for trans athletes and the duration of the levels in competition vary from organization to organization and have changed every couple of years for the last decade. In the sports world, there are numerous organizations—local, regional, and international. There are sports-specific as well as sports-general organizations. It is possible that there will be contradictory rules that are applicable to an athlete in two different organizations at the same time. Athletic organizations are striving for uniformity and consistency.

The IOC governs all Olympic sports in the world. Each country has its own Olympic organization, which follows the IOC's recommendations. The US Olympic Committee (USOC) is the national Olympic organization. In addition, each sport has its own national and international organizations. Two noteworthy organizations are the World Aquatics Organization (WAO), which is the international body of swimming, and the World Athletics Association (WAA), which is the international body of track and field. WADA is also involved. In the United States, the antidoping association is the USADA. Both organizations require TUEs for each drug an athlete may be taking, USADA for US events and WADA for international events.

The IOC and USOC have recommended each sports organization to develop its own sports-specific trans athlete policy. They have acknowledged that sports are different. Many sports organizations are in the process of writing these policies, and it has been observed that what makes a lot of sense in one sport may not in another. There are trans advocates who desire a universal trans policy that would include all sports, but this is unlikely at this time.

Cis females have a very low testosterone level unless they suffer from a medical condition such as PCOS. In fact, it is believed that if a cis female has a mildly elevated testosterone level, they probably have a mild DSD even if it is just PCOS. Testosterone is rarely elevated in cis female athletes, and low but abnormal levels of testosterone are often tolerated.

Trans females in the past have been allowed higher levels of testosterone than cis females. This is in part due to the difficulty in suppressing natural male testosterone levels. The number quoted for an ideal trans female testosterone level is often less than 55 ng/dL. The number depends on the organization quoted, and it can be higher. I have 40 years' experience in treating prostate cancer patients and know the acceptable castrate (removed testicles or on Lupron) testosterone level is less than 40 ng/dL. Neither modality may be affordable or available in parts of the United States and the world. Cyproterone acetate and spironolactone are used to suppress testosterone in most of the world but are not as predictable or reliable as castration or Lupron.

It seems that, given the difficulty in lowering testosterone, the levels chosen are a compromise value. Originally, the trans female testosterone level was set at 10 nmol/L, which is 288 ng/dL, a number often used as the lower limits of normal in cis males. A natural female level is about 40 ng/dL.

The sports organization numbers are currently all different and based on statistics and not scientific data. We are hopeful that uniformity in testosterone values will soon be achieved. The testosterone values for DSD athletes are also different when compared with trans athletes.

It is interesting and confusing to note that different organizations require different testosterone levels, and the levels may be different for trans women and for DSD women athletes. It is a point to remember that DSD testosterone states, while abnormal, are naturally occurring. The higher testosterone in the DSD athlete may be a medically necessary situation. It should also be remembered that it is often an all-or-nothing situation with testosterone. Lupron or castration may bring the level down to about 40 ng/dL, which is considered castrate. This level of testosterone in the castrated male comes from the adrenal glands. However, to lower testosterone to a specific level may not be possible. Lower testosterone in some DSDs may not be healthy.

Some organizations require DSD athletes to have a testosterone of 5 nmol/L. Recently, this number has been lowered to 2.5 nmol/L (72 ng/dL); although a more realistic number, it is easier said than done. This is as opposed to the trans female, who is usually allowed levels of 10 nmol/L or less. The duration of this low was two years; then it was lowered to one year, and now for some organizations it is six months. Inconsistencies defy common sense, and it is hoped that uniform standards will be established.

In some DSDs such as AIS, testosterone levels tend to be high, but this, of course, has no effect. It makes no sense to include all DSDs together but rather to evaluate the athlete on an individual basis with a checklist, which will be discussed later in the book.

Testosterone, Hemoglobin, and Hematocrit

Hemoglobin is the red blood cell pigment that carries oxygen. Hematocrit is the number of red blood cells. For our purposes, these two go hand in hand and are sometimes used interchangeably. When they are low, the patient is said to be anemic. Anemic people have diminished energy and diminished exercise capacity and are often short of breath. Higher hemoglobin and hematocrit can be of value for both aerobic and anaerobic exercises. There are several drugs that can be abused by athletes for an increase in hemoglobin and hematocrit, one of which is testosterone. The prototypic sport for abusing drugs to elevate one's hemoglobin and hematocrit is cycling.

When testosterone is lowered with Lupron to treat prostate cancer, a patient often becomes anemic and is short of breath. This reinforces the role of testosterone, hemoglobin, and hematocrit in athletic performance. The effects are rarely seen in adolescents because they are young and healthy and are able to tolerate a lower blood count. Women have 5–15% lower hemoglobin and hematocrit than men. While some of the reduction may be attributed to menstruation, the difference is also seen in postmenopausal and nonmenstruating women. This difference is believed to be due to testosterone.

Testosterone has multiple effects on the production of red blood cells. It works as a growth factor by itself. It increases the production of erythropoietin from the kidneys, which is a very strong hormone for the production of red blood cells. It also has several other effects including increasing the body's iron levels, which is necessary for hemoglobin production. In the absence of testosterone, other hormones have effects, although not as robust.

Most of the increase in the blood cell production in men is thought to be due to testosterone and androgen receptors. It is unknown if the Y chromosome alone or testosterone in the absence of androgen receptors plays a role. This is important because, if it is androgen receptor dependent, complete androgen insensitivity syndrome (CAIS) should be accompanied by anemia. Those with androgen insensitivity syndrome do not menstruate, which needs to be taken into consideration. In reality, hemoglobin and hematocrit levels are variable in CAIS.

There are many unknowns in the subjects of testosterone and red blood cells. Testosterone's effect on red blood cells needs to be considered in any discussion on testosterone's effect on performance.

Testosterone Safety in Trans Males

Is testosterone safe to take? How about for bodybuilders who want a super-high level? What about different forms of testosterone? Or synthetic androgens like those used in veterinary medicine?

It is believed that in standard formulations and doses, testosterone is safe, although it does require physician monitoring. Unusual formulations of high doses and supplementation in cis males who have subnormal levels or borderline levels are less clearly understood and may not be safe. Trans males are prescribed normal doses of normal formulations of testosterone. It should be noted that any formulation is generally expensive.

Testosterone has a number of side effects, some of which are desired in the trans male. Testosterone effects are more significant if given prepuberty and if estrogen is blocked with Lupron or a hysterectomy is performed. Desirable side effects for the trans male include facial hair, deepened voice, and increased muscular development. Undesired side effects may be an increased red blood cell mass, acne, and liver abnormalities. The increased red blood cells can result in blood clots in the legs and lungs, which would be a serious medical situation. A patient on testosterone must therefore be monitored closely.

A full transition takes two to six years of hormone therapy. Other drugs may be administered, such as Proscar to stop hair loss and aromatase inhibitors to stop gynecomastia (breast swelling). Blood levels of testosterone must be maintained at the appropriate sports organization level, and TUEs need to be in order. It is important to note that medicine is very much an art and not a science. The desirable effects of testosterone rarely correlate with the blood levels of the hormone, and the drug must be carefully titrated to the desired effect while keeping levels within the permissible range.

Testosterone-Level Chart

There is great variation and inconsistency as to what constitutes a normal testosterone level for various individuals. When the information was unclear, I used the levels that were used in my practice.

Conversion Chart

United States ng/dL   multiply (×) by 0.0347 = world nmol/L
World nmol/L   divide (/) by 0.0347 = United States ng/dL

World	United States
2.5 nmol/L	72 ng/dL
5 nmol/L	144 ng/dL
10 nmol/L	288 ng/dL

Natural Cis Levels

Cis Adult Male 250–1,000 ng/dL
Cis Male Puberty up to 1,250 ng/dL
Cis Male Prepuberty 40 ng/dL
Cis Male Castrated 40 ng/dL
Cis Adult Female 15–40 ng/dL
Cis Female Puberty 15–70 ng/dL
Cis Female Prepuberty 20 ng/dL

Trans

Trans Female less than 70 ng/dL
Trans Male less than 1,000 ng/dL

DSD

PCOS 140 ng/dL

AIS

ACH

5-ARD

Heterogenous group of diseases with variable testosterone levels.

This chart should only be used as a guide. If an athelete is competing in a sport, they need to know and follow the sports organization's rules and numbers.

5

The Reality of Gender Dysphoria

Transgender versus DSD

Most of the attention in this debate is given to trans individuals, who are people born one sex but identify as another. People often fail to recognize that a large part of the concern is in sports that involve DSD athletes. DSD athletes are individuals born with some difference in sexual development where they are not clearly male or female. They can be incompletely developed or have characteristics of more than one sex. The issue that comes up in sports is mainly about individuals who identify as female but have elevated testosterone levels. This is not uncommon, particularly in women's track and field. DSD athletes exist in every combination of genotypic sex with associated sexual identity, but the main ones that are of concern are genotypic males, XY, with female identities and elevated testosterone levels. The elevated testosterone level may be medically necessary for health and may not be arbitrarily lowered to a certain level. These athletes may also be on other medications that would require a TUE from WADA.

Attempts to assign a sex to these children based on their genotypic or phenotypic sex are often met with failure. This is particularly true in the more severe cases. These children's sexual identities are best achieved by letting the child choose as they age. They generally know what sex they are by the age of six and often as early as two. Classical DSDs occur in 1 in 1,000 to 1 in 5,000 live births, depending on what one classifies as a DSD. Sometimes much lower numbers are quoted because they include other diagnoses as DSDs that are not classically included. Gender dysphoria occurs as frequently as 6 in 1,000 births. DSDs will be discussed in detail in future chapters. The existence of DSDs is used by some people as medical evidence of gender dysphoria.

Identity versus Orientation

Are transgender people gay? Transgender people have a gender identity mismatch. They feel and express themselves differently than their genotypic gender. We all think of XY cis males who become XY trans females and create controversy in women's athletics. While trans females are slightly more common or at least more spoken about than trans males, there is a significant number of XX females who identify as trans males. They are also involved in men's athletics. There is a false belief that they are less competitive against cis males and therefore come under less scrutiny. While this may be the case in very high-level sports, it is not universally true. There are certainly isolated incidences of trans males beating cis males.

Sexual orientation is the gender or sex that an individual is attracted to. Its point of reference is the gender identity of the person for whom there is an attraction, not their biological sex. This can be very confusing. If a cis male is attracted to a cis female, they are heterosexual. If a cis or trans male is attracted to a cis or trans female, they are still heterosexual. If a cis or trans male is attracted to a cis or trans male, they are gay. If a cis or trans female is attracted to a cis or trans female, they are lesbian. Remember, gender identity is what you go to bed as, and sexual orientation is who you go to bed with.

The answer to the question of trans people's sexual orientation is actually simple. It can be heterosexual or homosexual. It can also be bisexual, pansexual, or asexual. The thing to remember is that the orientation is referenced to the identity.

If transgender and gay people are not the same, then why are they included in the initials LGBTQ? It is not because they are the same but because of the power in numbers.

Nature versus Nurture

There is continuing controversy in medicine as to whether disease or behavior is caused by genes (nature) or by the environment (nurture). It is good to start with a biological example such as cancer, specifically lung cancer. It is well accepted that smoking causes lung cancer. It is also known that certain genetic defects predispose people to lung cancer. The majority of people with lung cancer, at a young age, have a genetic defect. Many of them also have tobacco exposure even with secondhand smoke. This is known as the two-hit hypothesis. It is said that your genes load the gun, but your lifestyle pulls the trigger. If someone has one of the genes that predisposes them to lung cancer but has a very healthy lifestyle, they may not get lung cancer. On the other hand, someone who does not have the gene but is a heavy smoker may still get lung cancer. These are two variables that are intertwined, nature and nurture. Continue reading to get an understanding of how gender identity is influenced by both nature and nurture.

Twin Studies

The concept of nature versus nurture works very well in areas other than medical conditions like lung cancer. It explains some of the origins of psychiatric disorders such as schizophrenia. It also partly explains variations in sexual orientation such as homosexuality. This is not to suggest that there is anything psychopathological about gay people; it just helps to suggest an origin of some behavior that may be hard to explain otherwise.

There was a time when an alternative sexual orientation was classified as a psychological disorder, but with a better understanding of the frequency and universality, it was accepted. It was moved to being a normal alternative lifestyle. Gender dysphoria is still a diagnosable condition, according to the American Psychiatric Association. In the past, they classified it as a disorder, but recently there has been a movement to classify it as an alternative norm. It comes up as a psychiatric classification because of dysphoria or the discomfort caused by it. More on this is discussed later. At this point, this is good because of the funds required for medications and surgical procedures. While it is hoped that all health insurance will treat gender dysphoria in the future, it is believed that it will be moved from a psychiatric classification to a congenital medical condition and eventually just an alternative norm.

Schizophrenia is an example of a psychiatric disorder that has both a nature and nurture component to it. The lung cancer example is easy for most people to understand, whereas psychological/psychiatric problems are a little more difficult. In schizophrenia, there is a genetic component and an environmental component. This is illustrated by twin studies.

Identical twins have the same DNA. One sperm fertilizes one egg, and in early development, they split into two embryos, hence two infants with identical DNA. The nature is identical. If raised in the same family, the nurture is very similar. If put up for adoption, the nurture is different. While separately adopted identical twins with schizophrenia are rare, they have been studied and support the nature-versus-nurture argument.

If both twins have the disorder, it is said to be concordant. If one has it and the other does not, it is discordant. The concordant rate for identical twins raised in the same household is approximately 50% for schizophrenia. When they are raised in different households as in the case of adoption, it is clearly lower, although it is difficult to cite an exact number. If the twins are nonidentical, born from two eggs and two sperm, they are siblings, different in nature but close to identical in nurture because they are raised together. The nonidentical twins' concordant rate is approximately 15%. All of this can be confusing, but it illustrates a strong, although incomplete, genetic component of schizophrenia.

What about something like sexual orientation? Does same-sex attraction have a genetic component? The simple answer is yes, and in twin studies on homosexuality, as many as 66% of identical and 30% of nonidentical twins are concordant for homosexuality. The number drops when they are raised in separate households. This suggests both a genetic and an environmental role in its origin. It needs to be made clear that there is no identified gene for homosexuality (queer gene). It is only deduced by twin studies and the high incidence of concordance. Since no specific gene is identified, it may very well be polygenetic, involving more than one gene. Let us not forget that nurture plays an important role.

Trans Twins

It can be seen from the discussion of concordance and identical twins that numerous medical, psychological, and social situations have both a genetic nature and an environmental nurture (nature versus nurture) component to them.

How does gender dysphoria fit in? It is still classified as a psychological problem when it results in distress, although it is no longer classified as a disorder by itself. It may require medical treatment and has many social implications. Is there an inherent component to gender identity and the associated dysphoria? The research on this subject is in its infancy, but the identical twin concordance rate is estimated at 25%, and the nonidentical rate is 5%. Some more recent studies focusing on US children in adolescence and male-to-female trans individuals have come up with twin concordance rates of over 60% for birth assigned males and 40% for birth assigned females. This data is still early and is not fully verified. Recall that identical twin concordance for gay people is 66%, and the nonidentical rate is 30%. I have had both concordant twins and siblings with gender dysphoria in my practice.

The early studies suggest a genetic component as well as an environmental component to gender identity dysphoria. Some theories suggest that in utero hormone levels affect the fetus's neurologic development. It is felt that in the future, some genetic markers will be identified that are associated with gender dysphoria. Despite a strong concordance rate in gay and lesbian twins, no genetic markers have been identified to date. Schizophrenia, on the other hand, has several associated genes. A medical condition such as lung cancer has several possible genetic abnormalities. Only time will tell where gender dysphoria fits in.

Crossdressers and Drag Queens

It is important to remember that there are almost as many trans males as there are trans females. Researchers believe that the actual number of trans males is greater than reported and that they fall under the radar. This is because trans males have an easier time adapting to society and assuming a male identity. Trans male children have always been accepted and been classified as "tomboys." Nobody ever discusses trans male athletes because they are successful at a much lower rate in most sports, although this may in part be a myth.

Crossdressers and the archaic medical term *transvestites* have nothing to do with gender dysphoria in trans females. As stated earlier in the definitions section, this is an individual, usually heterosexual, who derives some thrill from dressing as a woman. It can actually be classified as a type of fetish. It can also be a woman who dresses as a man. They tend to overdress and stand out, whereas a trans female tries to assume the gender appearance of the sex they identify with—a female. The trans person tries not to stand out or attract attention. They just strive for the appearance of the sex they identify with. They attempt to achieve a gender presentation that is as close to cis female or cis male as possible. Their goal is to be "passable" and to have no one suspect that they are anything but female. There are actually female crossdressers, too, but they mostly go unnoticed.

Drag queens are part of a long tradition of gay performers, often with a degree of comedy. They have nothing to do with trans people. The gay community often has mixed feelings about their behavior, particularly with the recent publicity they have received.

Trans women have a difficult time assuming the appearance of a woman and are often confused with crossdressers and drag queens. Some of this is done deliberately to detract from what most medical personnel feel is a real situation. The confusion about and criticism of drag queens are often perpetuated by anti-trans activists.

Trans People in Other Cultures

Gender identity exists in the animal kingdom. There are many examples of transgender and homosexual behavior observed in animals. Throughout history, trans individuals and groups have been documented in society; though sometimes accepted, they are more often persecuted.

There are at least half a dozen contemporary societies that recognize and accept or tolerate a third or fourth sex/gender. Some are understood to be transient in youth, although these often are accepted as permanent. Some of this includes DSDs. There are an unknown number of these cultures because many of the trans individuals are persecuted.

Because there are apparently transient trans behaviors in some societies, it supports the concept of not doing any major irreversible surgery to the individual until they are an adult. There is also a need for thorough evaluation of these individuals. Lupron is not considered medically permanent. It needs to be restated that in the United States, transient gender dysphoria is rare, and the detransition rate is thought to be under 3%.

More often than not, transgender individuals along with homosexuals are rejected, persecuted, and even executed in less liberal societies. This has been particularly true of athletes.

Detransitioning/Desistance

Desistance is the technical word for detransitioning, although it is rarely used. There are not a lot of quality studies on trans individuals because much of the gender-confirmation surgery is done privately and not in well-established programs. The surgery is also performed in Eastern Europe and the Far East. It has not been done for more than 50 years and is often done secretively. Transitioning involves three parts: presentation, hormones, and, ultimately, surgery. If somebody were to detransition after presentation, it would go unnoticed. If after hormones, it would not be completely obvious. If after surgery, there would be anatomic changes. It is thought that the number of detransitions may be low because it is underreported, and people are embarrassed to admit to it.

In high-quality studies with well-established programs, which include psychiatric support and a delay in surgery, detransition incidents are estimated at 1–3%. This is in both children and adults. This is the accepted rate in quality medical literature. Recent reports estimating rates of 15–20% are attributed to low-quality studies and case reports (one-person stories) as well as foreign studies. However, the 15–20% has been seized by the media and used as an argument against transitioning. It is important to take all of this data seriously. If the detransitioning rate is 15–20%, there should be a moratorium on transitioning. This is not the case in the view of organized medicine.

It is important to note that the detransitioning rate is

slightly higher in autistic children and adolescents. It is also slightly higher with the associated diagnosis of depression. This is, of course, a concern, but high-quality studies do not feel this number is significant.

Medicine's Acceptance of Gender Dysphoria

Just 10 years ago, most medical organizations were indecisive about and often opposed on paper to gender dysphoria issues. It has become clear that these issues are common, medically and psychologically real, and can result in serious harm to the individual, often a child or young adult, if not addressed. Current policy by most organizations including pediatric and urological societies is that the patient needs to be accepted and treated. However, there are states with politically motivated medical societies and individuals who oppose and deny the reality of gender dysphoria and limit its treatment.

One must separate the issue of gender dysphoria with the associated hormone and surgical treatment from issues involving trans athletes. The two are not the same thing. No medical person should deny the existence of gender dysphoria and trans people, but many feel that trans athlete issues are yet to be resolved.

The problem with trans athlete issues is that they have become highly politicized, which has affected the medical, hormonal, and surgical treatment of these individuals. Medical issues are best treated by a medical person and not by politicians. This has been the source of difficulty with other socially related issues such as abortion and most recently

COVID-19. Once society accepts that gender dysphoria and trans individuals are a reality that is not going away, they can then deal with the trans athlete.

American Psychiatric Society's Classification of Gender Dysphoria

The American Psychiatric Society publishes the *Diagnostic and Statistical Manual of Mental Disorders* (*DSM*) for the classification of all psychiatric and behavior-related disorders, including gender dysphoria. In the past, the *DSM* classified gender dysphoria as a disorder. This can be confusing, but a disorder is akin to a disease. In the last edition of the *DSM-5*, they changed *gender dysphoria disorder* to *gender dysphoria*. It is no longer classified as a disorder but rather as a situation that can cause emotional distress and depression and does require treatment. It gives a separate diagnostic code for both adults and children. This is acceptance by the medical community of the reality of gender dysphoria without the classification of it as a disease. The fact that there are diagnostic codes for a condition makes it a legal medical diagnosis and allows insurance to pay for patient treatments.

6

Differences (Disorders) in Sexual Development

Introduction

Differences in sexual development, which were formerly known as disorders of sexual development, occur at variable rates depending on what one classifies as a DSD. As mentioned earlier, DSDs comprise over 60 different syndromes. There is no universal agreement in medicine as to which disorders or differences should be characterized as a DSD. The thing that characterizes all the disorders or differences, however, is the confusion of the child's sex— confusion between the genetic or chromosomal sex and the appearance of the child's genitals. Most of these syndromes are too complicated for our discussion. It is, however, beneficial to study some of the common syndromes because they can help us understand some of the controversies involving testosterone and trans athletes.

The literature lists the incidences of classic DSDs as anywhere from 1 in 1,000 to 1 in 5,000. More recent numbers have listed the incidences of DSDs as 0.5 in 1,000. The reason for this wide variation in the occurrence of DSDs has to do with what is included. Some studies include chromosomal abnormalities, and some do not. Some include PCOS, which is very common. Perhaps the largest discrepancy exists with minor anomalies of secondary sexual characteristics. This includes individuals with undescended testes, which are testes that are not in the scrotum. It also includes hypospadias, or abnormalities of the pee hole on the penis. These anomalies are very common, and if these individuals are counted, the numbers increase greatly. If one were to include only classic DSDs, which are listed in the following pages, with the exception of PCOS, the incidence rate is more in the 1 in 1,000 to 1 in 5,000 range, as mentioned above. It should also be noted that some recent studies have allowed self-reporting, and this has further confused the numbers.

DSDs are nature's experiment in gender identity. Healthcare providers who treat DSDs have learned an important lesson. The lesson is that gender is complex and cannot be confused with genotypic or phenotypic sex. Gender is a combination of chromosomes, genes, hormones in utero, appearance, and rearing. Gender cannot be assigned by a third-party healthcare provider. When there is some confusion, the child's input is essential.

Children born with more severe DSDs may require a period of growth, usually two to six years, to establish their own gender identity. When I treated such patients, the team would explain to the parents that the child was born prematurely in the sex department and that they may require a little time to define their sex. This was difficult for the parent to handle, particularly in the past, but today it has become much more acceptable to the family and is less embarrassing.

The fact that there is such a thing as a DSD and that they can have gender dysphoria adds credibility to the reality of gender dysphoria. The cause of gender dysphoria still remains unknown, and while there can be multiple causes, there is some evidence of a genetic etiology. This goes against the political beliefs that gender dysphoria is a transient social phenomenon.

As mentioned, there is thought to be an incident rate of 1 in 1,000 to 1 in 5,000 for classic DSDs. The incidence of gender dysphoria in this group is variable depending on which DSD but is thought to be approximately 30%. DSDs are pediatric neonatal diagnoses, and for that reason, gender dysphoria in this group is often underreported. An understanding of DSD can lead to a better understanding of gender dysphoria.

It is worth mentioning again that DSDs occur in the animal kingdom. The less complex an organism is, the more common and extreme intersex issues are. Humans are complex organisms and do not tolerate anything more than simple genetic anomalies. Many of the anomalies that exist in the animal kingdom might be fatal in humans.

Commonly Encountered DSDs

The following is a list of DSDs commonly encountered in athletes. Chromosomal abnormalities can be considered a DSD but rarely show up in sports. Most DSDs have a genetic component even if the genes are unknown. Some of the DSDs have no effect on hormones or performance. The problem occurs when an athlete of either gender identity, usually female, has an elevated testosterone level. It is believed by some that any athlete genetically male or female with an elevated testosterone level, without the presence of a testosterone-producing tumor, has an undiagnosed subclinical DSD. Depending on which disorders are included as DSDs, the incidences may be gravely underestimated. This list is in the order of the most common to the least common classic DSDs.

1. Polycystic ovary syndrome (PCOS)—not universally accepted as a DSD
2. Adrenal cortical hyperplasia (ACH) / adrenal genital syndrome (AGS)
3. Androgen insensitivity (AI) / testicular feminization syndrome: Complete (CAI), partial (PAI), mild (MAI)
4. 5-alpha reductase deficiency (5-ARD)
5. Ovotestis syndrome

Polycystic Ovary Syndrome

PCOS, also known as Stein Leventhal syndrome, is not universally accepted as a DSD, but with an increased testosterone level, it has been the cause of drug-test failures and must be addressed. The incidence is 1 in 500 to 1 in 1,000. These adolescents at the time of puberty have an imbalance of their pituitary and ovary hormones, which produce too much testosterone. Levels can be as high as

130–150 ng/dL. This is enough to fail a drug test. They also have insulin resistance and tend to be overweight. The increased testosterone causes acne and hirsutism (body/facial hair). Alopecia (hair loss) can also occur. The treatment involves Glucophage, diabetes medications, or spironolactone (an antiandrogen diuretic), which requires a TUE. It may not be so simple to decrease testosterone to an acceptable level, which is currently often 2.5 nmol/L. This DSD tends to show in power sports like softball and weightlifting. While this tends to masculinize the people with it, it has an inconsistent effect on sexual identity, and most studies show little or no increase in incidence of gender dysphoria. PCOS is thought to be the common reason for elevated testosterone in young women. Some sports organizations discount PCOS regardless of the testosterone levels. The reason that it is often not included as a DSD is the mild elevation of testosterone and the XX, female genotype.

Adrenal Cortical Hyperplasia

ACH, also known as AGS, Adrenal Genital Syndrome, is believed to be the most common of the true DSDs if one counts both XX and XY together. This is the most common XX DSD. True DSDs are those with abnormal genitalia or significant hormone abnormalities. This is an autosomal recessive condition, which means that affected individuals get one gene from each parent. The parent may be an asymptomatic carrier, have a mild form of the disease, or even have the full-blown disease. This condition may or may not cause infertility depending on its severity and associated medications that need to be taken. Today, with assisted reproductive technology, many patients with DSDs can achieve fertility, whereas they may not have been able to in the past. The incidence of this is estimated to be greater than 1 in 5,000 live births. With this condition, the affected individual lacks an enzyme in the adrenal gland that makes mineral corticoids. Mineral corticoids are hormones such as aldosterone. This is a cortisone-like hormone that stops the loss of salt in the urine. Ninety-five percent of these cases are a deficiency of 21-hydroxylase, and since it is the most common form, it is the only one that we will discuss in detail.

The body is able to detect the shortage of aldosterone and, in order to compensate, ramps up the production of all other adrenal cortical hormones. This results in increased levels of sex hormones, which are predominantly androgen (testosterone). Recall that the adrenal cortex makes cortisone, aldosterone, and sex hormones, which are predominantly androgens.

This syndrome occurs in both men and women. In genetic males, XY, it is often insignificant in adulthood and may only be a salt-losing problem or a blood pressure dehydration problem in infancy. In a mild form, it may go unnoticed or may result in an adult with mildly elevated testosterone levels. More often, an adult male may be on aldosterone or cortisone, and if he is an athlete, he will require a TUE.

Uniquely, the cis male with high testosterone may have precocious (early) puberty and may have premature effusion of their epiphysis (growth plates), resulting in a short stature. This might give them an advantage in a sport like weightlifting, but this has never been addressed in the literature that I am aware of.

The problem with the condition that occurs is in the genetic female (XX). The high levels of androgens (testosterone) result in masculinization/ambiguity of their genitalia and a phenotypic male sexual appearance. Besides needing mineral corticoids and cortisone, for which a TUE would be involved, they may also have higher-than-normal levels of testosterone or one of the other adrenal androgens. The testosterone, which would be functional, could improve their athletic performance. This is what causes controversy in sports medicine. These individuals do have gender dysphoria above the level of cis females. To compete in an athletic event, the athlete will need to have a DSD-approved testosterone level, which is easier said than done because exact titration of testosterone levels is quite difficult.

It is believed that these athletes are involved in multiple sports including track and field. They argue against the necessity of changing the testosterone level when it is a naturally occurring state and not by choice. Defenders of athletes cite social, political, and human rights issues in their defense. DSD athletes are such a varied group that it is becoming clear that they need to be evaluated on an individual basis, just as the sport needs to establish its own individual rules.

Like most DSDs in children, ACH is diagnosed and treated at infancy. Besides medical/hormonal treatment, surgical treatment may be necessary. It is estimated that there is approximately a 15% incidence of gender dysphoria in this disorder. Because of the high amount of androgens in utero, there is a tendency for XX girls to have a male identity. The reason for such a relatively low incidence of gender dysphoria, when compared with some of the other DSDs, is thought to be relatively early hormone and surgical intervention if necessary.

Moreover, 17-hydroxylase deficiency and 11-hydroxylase deficiency are two of several other enzyme deficiencies in the other 5% that are not 21-hydroxylate deficiency ACH. They are usually severe disorders; 17-hydroxylase results in XY males with no virilization because of a complete lack of androgens, while 11-hydroxylase is a more severe form of 21-hydroxylase, which usually involves masculinized females. The 17- and 11-hydroxylase deficiencies have significant gender identity issues compared with the 21-hydroxylase. Part of the low incidence of gender dysphoria in 21-hydroxylase is that it is recognized in infancy and treated with hormones and surgery. The 17-hydroxylase deficiency, which has almost no androgens in utero and as infants, has a uniform female gender identity despite an XY genotype. This suggests the role of hormones intrauterine in gender identity. These children have little male genital development and are usually converted into females in infancy. That is why 17-hydroxylase deficiency, which is a severe DSD, is used as an example of why children should be treated earlier in life.

Androgen Insensitivity Syndrome

AIS, also known as testicular feminization, occurs in three broad categories: complete (CAIS), partial (PAIS), and mild forms (MAIS). Its incidence is 2–5 per 100,000 for the complete form. PAIS has a similar incidence but can be undiagnosed, and the numbers are uncertain. Mild forms of AIS are common and thought to be the cause of minor genitourinary anomalies in male infants. This is an oversimplification, and in reality, there are over 100 different forms of this disease described with different genetic inheritance.

The individuals are XY and either lack or have a defective androgen or testosterone receptor on their cells. The hormone testosterone can be thought of as the key and the receptor as the lock. If the lock is missing its keyhole or has a different keyhole, the key cannot work. In this case, none of the testosterone function is "opened" or "unlocked."

It is often diagnosed with an adolescent girl who fails to menstruate or when a child or adolescent girl has a hernia repair, and the hernia is found to contain undescended testes. The undescended testes have a high risk of becoming a malignant tumor, and with CAIS, they are removed. In other parts of the world, this is not always the case. With PAIS, if the child is being raised as a male, the testes can be left until after the child goes through natural puberty, and then the testes can be removed. If the PAIS child is being raised as a female, they can be removed as soon as they are discovered.

Complete Androgen Insensitivity Syndrome

This is straightforward because the people who have it have a female phenotype. The testosterone they have does nothing. They look female, and there is no one who would dispute they are female in an athletic contest. They have a delay in puberty, and they tend to be a little taller than the average female their age. The testosterone is broken down to estrogen so that they develop as a female. Anti-trans activists note that they are still a little taller and have a Y chromosome. The role of the Y chromosome in the absence of testosterone or testosterone receptors is unknown. There are also concerns regarding their blood count.

Partial Androgen Insensitivity Syndrome

The affected individuals have one of several defects in the androgen receptor "lock" and do not fully masculinize or develop as men. They often have ambiguous genitalia, leading them toward surgery if they want to become more male or female in appearance. People with CAIS usually have a female gender identity, but those with PAIS can be more variable in their appearance and have more gender dysphoria. CAIS identifies with the female gender because their androgens are functionless. This illustrates the importance of inutero hormones for gender identity. This is unlike people with PAIS, who can identify as either sex.

Theoretically, the testosterone levels in both syndromes, PAIS and CAIS, are higher than normal. The diagnosis is often known before any female child fails a drug test for high testosterone. They are usually diagnosed as phenotypic females with delayed puberty and no menstruation. In reality, the testosterone level in these individuals can be high or low for complex reasons, but what is consistent is a phenotypic female with high testosterone and an XY chromosome.

This can be a point of contention in sports medicine. These girls/women are phenotypically female but have a Y chromosome and testosterone. The concern is that even though they are female and lack the receptors for testosterone, they are deriving some benefit from the chromosome and the testosterone.

It is generally believed that with CAIS, this is not the case. However, those with PAIS are likely deriving some benefit. For that reason, there is a desire to have those with CAIS conform to DSD testosterone levels. Those with MAIS are usually identified as males and may rarely have testosterone levels elevated enough to create an issue. MAIS is discussed more in the section on policy.

There are still people who feel that high testosterone levels in these individuals can affect neurologic development, hemoglobin, and hematocrit (red blood cell number). Given the spectrum of AIS, it would require an evaluation of each on an individual basis to accurately assess the athlete.

5-Alpha Reductase Deficiency

5-ARD is one of over 60 DSDs. It was incorrectly thought to be relatively rare in the past. It needs to be mentioned because even though less common than some other DSDs, it is overrepresented in female-gender-identity DSD athletes. One of the reasons it is impossible to know the exact instances of a DSD like this in athletes is because medical records are confidential. In other parts of the world, there is often not enough sophistication to make some of these diagnoses, and these patients could possibly go undiagnosed unless they come up against a sports organization.

Testosterone is the main hormone responsible for athletic performance. This is discussed throughout the book. Humans have an enzyme called 5-alpha reductase that converts the testosterone to dihydrotestosterone, which is the hormone responsible for male secondary sex characteristics, including genital growth. Women have this enzyme, but it has little effect with the small amount of naturally occurring testosterone they have.

There are several syndromes of partial or near-complete genetic deficiencies of this enzyme that occur in small groups around the world. In these populations, there are usually three sexes—boys, girls, and girls who may or may not turn into boys or masculinize at the time of puberty. This occurs at puberty, when the testosterone level increases. Even though there is a deficiency of this enzyme, the testosterone is so high at puberty that even trace amounts of the enzyme can cause changes. Most of the time, these individuals become masculine girls with undescended testes.

These individuals are XY genotype. They appear phenotypically to be female, as with AIS. Unlike AIS, their testosterone is functional and can affect performance. Initially, when discussed, these individuals were incorrectly classified as having AIS. This makes older studies and the literature on these subjects very confusing.

5-alpha reductase is the enzyme that the drug Proscar blocks to stop hair loss and prostate growth in developed males. It has no effect on genital development after puberty is complete. The drug spironolactone also acts on 5-alpha reductase, and this is why it can be used to prevent testosterone-related hair loss.

People with 5-ARD are a heterogenous group depending on the degree of enzyme mutation. Most appear to be phenotypically female but are rather muscular. Testosterone is present, but the function is lower. The current recommended testosterone level for DSD athletes is 2.5 nmol/L to compete with cis female athletes. This is controversial because many have gone through a male puberty. There is thought to be about a 50% incidence of gender dysphoria in this group. The occurrence is thought to be common in women's track and field, and it creates a real challenge for the sports medicine community. The majority of occurrences is autosomal recessive, making them more common in ethnically isolated groups. However, they occur worldwide.

Ovotestis Syndrome

Formerly known as the "true hermaphrodite," this syndrome is a rare DSD, but it is included to help explain how complex biology can be. A child can be born with a mosaic of XX/XY chromosomes, thus having two sexes. Although rare in humans, it does occur and illustrates how complex gender can be. This person is born with two sexes and two genders. Given enough time, they will decide which gender identity they feel more comfortable as. Their gonads (ovaries and testes) often need to be removed because of the high incidence of cancer. When and which set or if both sets of gonads should be removed is a controversial subject. If the child identifies with a particular sex early, it may be possible to leave one set and allow the natural puberty and possibly monitor the gonads for cancer. The gonads can then be removed at a later date. It is clear that a child needs to develop their own identity, and past attempts to default the infant's sex to female were only about 50% successful. This illustrates the theme that gender is not single and fixed but binary and fluid. This is the most extreme example of a DSD.

Is Gender Dysphoria a DSD?

When I was a student and first became familiar with gender dysphoria, I logically assumed it was like a DSD, knowing that DSD patients had gender identity problems (often different from their genotypic sex). Like other people before me, I logically assumed that they were similar disorders. It was thought to be due to hormone effects or a neurological development in the brain or something to do with how children with DSDs were raised because of their ambiguous genitalia. There is some evidence of gender identity being affected by in utero hormones, and in addition, the role of nurture in many disorders cannot be discounted. One must remember that DSDs are a diverse group of disorders. Gender identity depends on the DSD, rearing, and phenotypic sex appearance. Many people with DSDs are treated at infancy.

At this point, gender dysphoria is not considered a DSD, but approximately 30% of those with DSDs have gender dysphoria. DSD athletes may show up in a sport as female with elevated testosterone.

It seems that gender dysphoria and gender identity in DSD athletes are very variable because of the many different DSDs. Many people still feel that gender dysphoria is created by intrauterine hormones, phenotypic appearance, early surgery, and natural or artificial hormones in their rearing. Some of these variables are naturally occurring, and some are medical and social interactions. Advocates for treating trans children feel that if the same options available to DSD children were available to gender dysphoric children, we would have less depression in younger adults with gender dysphoria than we do. There is good evidence to support this.

Half of the discussion on gender identity involves trans people and half those with DSDs. People with DSDs are a diverse group, some with chromosomal abnormalities, some with genetic syndromes (as outlined in the DSD section), and some with minor developmental anomalies of the genitals. There is not a complete agreement as to what counts as a DSD.

If we break the DSDs down into different subgroups, we have differences in gender identity among the various groups. For example, those with CAI whose androgens have no effect and are phenotypically female have very low gender dysphoria when raised as a female, whereas those with 5-ARD, which masculinizes at puberty, have approximately 50% gender dysphoria regardless of which sex they are raised as. It seems that the more phenotypically developed the DSD is, the less gender identity there is.

When someone is born with severe or confusing DSD, they are often not assigned a sex at birth but are given time to work out their own gender identity. Many problems are resolved both surgically and hormonally in DSD children. This may be why we hear less about DSD problems in adults. This is used as an argument for treating gender dysphoria early in children.

DSDs outside the United States

In the United States, there is legal opposition to the medical and surgical treatment of gender dysphoria. There is, however, no opposition to the treatment of children with DSD, even when it involves puberty-delaying drugs and gender-confirmation surgery. This is because DSD is recognized as a medically occurring abnormality with potential health risks. Examples are electrolytes and blood pressure problems with ACH and gonadal degeneration into malignancies with several different DSDs.

Medicine in the United States, compared with other parts of the world, is generally more sophisticated. In fact, many foreign doctors have trained in the United States. DSDs in the United States are treated by multidisciplinary teams with extensive family education and informed consent. The family is helped to understand the outcomes of treatment even if it is not as planned. Services like this are often not available in most countries.

The American medical community has learned, partly through prior errors, that people with severe DSDs need to establish their own gender identity before any radical permanent surgery is performed. We have also learned that certain DSDs are almost always aligned with a particular gender, and corrective surgery can be performed early in the child's life.

In many parts of the world, people with gender dysphoria are persecuted and mistreated. Both the United Nations (UN) and the World Health Organization (WHO) have come out as supporters of trans individuals, although it is unclear what effect it has had worldwide. These organizations basically see it as a human rights issue.

Many people are surprised to discover that the UN and the WHO are opposed to intersex treatment and surgery. They use the term *intersex,* not *DSD. DSD* is generally a preferred term in the United States.

What are the reasons for this position? Most of their objections to treatment, particularly surgery, are based on human rights issues because of lack of informed consent. Many other countries just do not have the support and programs we do in the United States. In some parts of the world, medicine can be much more authoritative. There rarely is parental education. The quality of surgery can also be inferior. This is usually not because of training but because of fewer facilities and little ancillary support. Results of the treatment of DSDs in children are far from perfect in the United States, but it is significantly worse in most of the rest of the world.

There have been cases where a child with a severe DSD was converted to a male gender at the patient's family's request only to grow up with a female gender identity. If time was taken with this severe DSD case, the child could have had female gender-confirmation surgery with better results. Ironically, the female gender would have been easier to establish.

Some of the worldwide objections to intersex treatment are because of female circumcision. Female circumcision is an archaic surgical procedure performed in many cultures and is condemned by all organized medical and human rights groups. Female circumcision is some variation of surgical clitorectomy and vaginal closure designed to eliminate orgasm and prevent sexual activity until marriage. It is battery and mutilation. Unfortunately, many variations of this surgical procedure are very similar to DSD surgeries, and there is confusion worldwide between female circumcision and DSD surgery. Both the UN and WHO have, along with other human rights issues, condemned DSD surgery because of this confusion.

Most of this is a misunderstanding, but it is also due to a lack of resources, both medically and socially. Advocates for people with DSDs worldwide focus on consent issues and realize that it is probably better to let these people grow up intersex and choose their gender-confirmation surgery as an adult when they are able to make better choices. While this view has some merit, it discounts the medical issues such as testicular and ovarian cancer, which can develop in adolescents and can be fatal.

More education is needed worldwide, as it is in the United States, before we can understand, accept, and appropriately treat transgender individuals and people with DSDs.

7

The History of Trans/DSD Athletes

The modern era of gender dysphoria and transgender surgery began in the 1940s, post World War II, with Christine Jorgensen. Christine is credited with being the first widely known trans woman. She underwent early sexual reassignment surgery, which is what it was called at the time, in Copenhagen, Denmark. The first of several surgeries was in 1952. Details and end results of her surgery are unknown, but it was claimed to be very successful. She was an instant celebrity but also partly a curiosity. She lived until 1989 and was a successful actress.

The history of trans/DSD athletes in organized sports has been contradictory and therefore confusing. An attempt is made here to supply a brief history.

It is difficult to estimate the numbers of trans/DSD individuals in the world. Admission of being trans or even homosexual in certain cultures can be a death sentence. In the United States, 1.6 million individuals identify as trans. The number with DSD is greater, although only about one-third of DSD patients have gender-dysphoria issues. They still have hormone irregularities and participate in organized sports. The histories of trans and DSD athletes are intermittently entwined, and it is difficult to separate one history from the other.

Current medical practices and legal precedence in many Western countries, particularly the United States, allow an individual to determine their gender by simply declaring what sex they are. Most of this is a matter of civil rights and human rights. Many critics of this policy feel that we are altering commonsense notions to accommodate progressive social ideas. Extreme views like this one, however, are not only inconsistent with developing medical knowledge but are disruptive because they close the dialogue on the subject. This will need to be followed over time to see how these issues develop.

Ever since the 1936 Berlin Olympics, officials have believed that Eastern European Soviet bloc athletes have been attempting to cheat the system by allowing men to compete as women. With the discovery of the Barr body in the 1960s, it became possible to check for this. The first time the Barr body was used in the Olympics was in 1968 in Mexico City. Officials were sure they would find numerous athletes who were Barr-body negative (genetic males) in the female division. They were surprised they found no cheaters, and the story goes that there was only one athlete identified without a Barr body in the female pool, but it was actually an athlete with DSD.

In 1975, tennis player Reneé Richards transitioned to a

female presentation. She wanted to play tennis in the US Open championship. She was already a fairly accomplished male tennis player. There was legal opposition, and she ultimately won a lawsuit that allowed her to play. When she was finally allowed to play, most of the competitors refused to compete with her.

An important point debated in trans athletics is strength versus skill. It, of course, depends on the sport. Trans females do not always win against cis females. Pro-trans-athlete advocates have argued that most men could not beat Serena Williams at tennis. Anti-trans advocates argue that "most" is not "all." All sports are different and need to be considered on an individual basis.

In Olympic sports, it is the individual sports organizations that decide their own policy. The IOC realizes that all sports are different and only makes recommendations, while the policies are determined by the individual sport. Whatever policy the IOC or the sports organization makes, it must be consistent with WADA's rules.

Prior to 2000, trans/DSD athletes were required to have chromosomal testing to prove their genetic sex. Initially, this was done by Barr body and was later replaced by karyotypes. It was soon realized that this was irrelevant because there were athletes with DSDs who were not clearly one sex or the other and fell more into a gender identity issue like a trans athlete. There were people with DSDs who were missing chromosomes or had extra chromosomes or mosaics. Sex or, more specifically, gender is not always chromosomal. A test like a Barr body, and subsequently karyotypes, was of limited value. In the distant past, athletes were subject to genital inspection to determine their appropriate sex, although this quickly fell out of favor.

In 2003, the IOC came up with a policy regarding trans athletes. They allowed trans athletes to compete if they legally changed their sex, had gender-confirmation surgery (removal of the testes if assigned male sex at birth), and had hormone levels for a two-year period that were consistent with the medically normal range of the sex they wished to compete as. Most of the policies addressed athletes who were male at birth, with the concern being mostly testosterone levels. In 2004, trans women were allowed to play in the Olympics.

In 2015, the IOC stopped requiring surgery because it was unavailable in many countries and because legal restrictions prohibited the surgery in other countries. Most of the concern was over athletes assigned male at birth. In general, athletes assigned female at birth had no restrictions as long as their testosterone levels were compatible with the cis male levels. It should be noted, however, that trans male athletes have only recently had their testosterone levels measured. Initially, they were just allowed to play with no testosterone measurements. Concerns about athletes with DSDs, particularly with a female gender identity and high testosterone, have only recently become an issue.

At the end of 2015 and the beginning of 2016, the IOC came up with a new policy on trans athletes. Most importantly, they recommended that each individual sport make its own policy. They abandoned the legal sex change, sex-confirmation surgery, and prolonged altered hormone levels.

In 2016, the IOC stated that "to require surgical and anatomic changes as a precondition to participation is no longer necessary to preserve fair competition and may be inconsistent with developing legislation and notions of human rights." After that statement, gender-confirmation surgery and a legal change of sex were no longer an issue. Hormone levels (testosterone) persisted as the main issue.

At the time, the IOC required testosterone levels to be consistent with the athlete's gender identity for one year prior to competition and throughout the competition. Initially, they only addressed trans females but subsequently included trans males and required a cis male level.

The prior lack of rules regarding trans females' testosterone levels was based on studies of one of the DSDs, ACH. Some early studies created the false belief that elevated testosterone levels in athletes were of limited value. There were also studies on CAIS, where testosterone has no effect. This led to a temporary erroneous belief that testosterone had little or no effect on athletic function. It should be noted that no trans athletes are believed to have competed in the 2016 Olympics, but several did in 2020.

In 2018, the IOC started to place testosterone-level restrictions on both trans females and trans males, including DSD athletes. WADA subsequently weighed in on this issue and has required trans athletes to have testosterone levels within a medically established range. For trans male athletes taking testosterone, the level of testosterone in their system must be within the normal cis male range, and they must have a TUE form on record. In addition, they must be on this medicine for a period of one year prior to playing.

Initially, the time duration of testosterone therapy was two years for some organizations, and a few organizations even required four years. Any other medications an athlete takes together with testosterone require a TUE.

Trans women often take estrogen replacement. Generally estrogens are not prohibited substances for antidoping purposes. An example of this would be birth control pills. There are several other drugs that the trans female athlete may be taking, including Lupron and spironolactone, to name a few. Estrogens work better with the addition of these medications to suppress the naturally occurring testosterone. A TUE should be obtained for these medications as they are on the WADA antidoping list. Currently, for trans female athletes, WADA requires them to have their testosterone level below 10 nmol/L, which is 288 ng/dL, although this is constantly changing and will likely be lowered to correspond to some other organizations' recommendations.

This information changes often with no advance notification. If anyone cares for a trans athlete, it is essential that they keep up with the rules; that includes sports medicine physicians, parents, and coaches. Information should ideally be posted on the sports organization, USOC, and USADA websites. A brief discussion of sports organization policy is included in future chapters. At the time of publication of this book, the policies are inconsistent, contradictory, and rapidly changing. Nothing in this book should be used as a reference; instead, the actual document should be cited. The purpose of this book is to provide background educational information. Statements and information in a book of this nature will be outdated by the time it is published.

8

Gender-
Confirmation
Surgery

Gender-confirmation surgery is the correct term. *Transgender surgery* is the second-best term. *Sex-change surgery* is incorrect and inappropriate. The trans person is not changing their sex but has surgery to help achieve their image of the gender they identify with. These terms can refer to various surgeries on different parts of the body performed separately or at the same time. Genital (bottom) surgery is often last because it is difficult, expensive, and requires prolonged recovery.

There was actually a time in sports when people thought it was necessary to change one's genital appearance to be recognized as the other sex. It has been stated over and over in this book that gender identity is what a person feels and identifies with, whether or not the genitals match their desired gender. In the United States and most of the Western world, someone is able to change their gender identity by simply declaring they are a certain gender. They can often apply for legal birth certificate changes after a certain time period. Hormones and surgery have nothing to do with the legality but are highly desired by the trans person in order to develop a full body image. All of the legal rules vary from locality to locality.

Initial (top) surgery for trans females includes hair removal, breast augmentation (implants), facial plastic surgery, thyroid cartilage shaving (Adam's apple), and other procedures designed to feminize the individual. Surgery for trans males includes bilateral mastectomies, liposuction, facial plastic surgery, and, possibly, a hysterectomy if children are not desired.

Even before or after the surgeries, the individual is on hormones and the associated drugs for a period of time. Trans males are on testosterone, and trans females are on estrogen. If they have not been surgically castrated by removing their testes or ovaries, they often need testosterone or estrogen suppression with a drug such as Lupron. They may also require other medications as listed in the drug section. A full hormone transition requires two to six years.

The treatment is conducted by a team of physicians. The primary care physician is often the coordinator. Hormones may require an endocrinologist or a pediatric endocrinologist. An endocrinologist is a hormone doctor. All programs should have a full psychiatric evaluation, although this is not always the case. The surgery is performed in part by a plastic surgeon and in part by a urologist. With DSD, a geneticist or developmental pediatrician may be part of the team.

A male-to-female gender-confirmation surgery is removal of the male genitals with creation of a neovagina between the anus and urethra (pee tube). The skin of the penis is inverted into a new vagina, and the scrotum is used to form labia. Packing (gauze) needs to remain in the neovagina for a week while the person is hospitalized. Subsequently, it needs to be dilated. Good function and orgasm are the rule with today's surgical techniques because the nerves of the penis are preserved.

In female-to-male gender-confirmation surgery, a neophallus (penis) is created by taking a muscle, including its artery and vein, usually from the forearm, and attaching it to the pubic bone just above the vagina, which is closed. The labia are fused into a scrotum, and two artificial (silicone) testes are inserted. The most difficult part of the surgery is creating a urethra to urinate through. This may take several operations and can have a high failure rate, forcing some patients to void through a hole in front of their anus. This is often disappointing because the true image of a male is standing to void, not sitting. At a later date, attempts can be made to revise the urethra, but results are still limited. A penile implant can also be inserted with reasonable results. The male-to-female is an easier and more successful operation than the female-to-male operation. This is true of all procedures where something is removed versus being added. This is the reason female-to-male surgery is performed less frequently. Many times, the entire trans male transformation is performed without the creation of a neophallus. To the nonmedical person, the description of the surgery sounds incredible, but it can be achieved with good plastic surgery results. Both sexes can be functional and achieve orgasm.

All of the secondary sex-characteristic surgeries are sometimes referred to as *top surgery* and the actual genital surgery as *bottom surgery*. Since the surgeries are available in other parts of the world as well as the United States, the results can be quite variable. In the United States, in experienced hands, the results of top surgery are excellent, and those for bottom surgery are as outlined above. Small revisions with future surgeries are necessary, and over 50% of trans female bottom surgeries have end results that are satisfactory. It is the trans male operation that has less satisfactory results because of its complexity, and it has led some surgeons to advocate for trans male top surgery only.

Results in less trained surgical hands are generally poor, and if an expert surgical team is not available, it may be better to avoid bottom surgery on both trans men and trans women. Remember that there are three parts to transitioning: presentation, hormones, and top and bottom surgery. The surgery is often the least important.

Do Minors Have a Right to Transition?

This has become a legal controversy in the United States and is usually subject to state laws, although there is a trend toward national legislation. In most states, the legal age to consent to surgery is usually 18, although there are states that allow 16- or 17-year-olds to consent. Parents can usually give consent for a minor, and in the case of a medical emergency such as appendicitis, it would be a crime if the parent did not procure surgical treatment for their child. In many states, elective plastic surgery can be performed on a child with the parent's consent. If the child has a deformity, it certainly should be repaired. What about an elective nose job? Children with DSDs often have operations with the acknowledgment that they may have gender identity issues in the future. This book is about medical controversies and not political or legal controversies, although the two are inseparable. This section is included as an introduction to a subject in order to stimulate thought.

One of the controversies involving surgery on minors is detransitioning (changing one's mind), which is generally very low, usually 1–3% of cases. There have been several TV documentaries about children and young adults who have changed their minds. These documentaries have a strong political agenda.

Opponents of child or adolescent gender dysphoria feel it is a psychiatric problem and requires counseling. They also oppose the puberty-blocking drugs such as Lupron. Opposition is due to the false belief that the drug is unsafe. Arguments are made that puberty may not resume once the drug is stopped. This is rare, and most people treated with Lupron go on to get gender-confirmation surgery, so this is not an issue. Other risks are osteoporosis, hip fractures, increased height, and perhaps some rare tumors. The drug is used extensively in adult males for prostate cancer and in females for gynecological issues, so there is a lot of experience with its side effects. Pediatric endocrinologists use it to increase the height of short-stature children and to delay puberty in children who are maturing too fast. The experience is generally good. Politically, people criticize the cost ($125 a month) and the spending of Medicaid/Medicare and other government monies. Failure to use puberty blockers in a prepubertal child prior to transition results in inferior transitioning outcomes. This is particularly true of testosterone's effects, which are hard to mitigate after puberty. If the concern is future athletic performance, it is the testosterone at puberty that will result in most of the advantages for the future trans female.

The consequences of not allowing the child to choose their own sexual identity include severe psychological maladjustment, depression, substance abuse, and suicidal thought. When trans individuals are supported as children, they thrive. If the medical community had a medical way to prevent adolescent depression and suicide, they would embrace it. Well, they do in this situation. All they need to do is support these trans children, even if there is political opposition to their treatment.

Proponents of trans children make an analogy with a disease like diabetes or cancer. It is the parent or guardians who must advocate for the child's health. Nobody would condone withholding medical treatment that works for children because they are under 18. In fact, a parent would be guilty of neglect and abuse if they denied medical care to a child. Gender dysphoria is classified by the American Psychiatric Association's *DSM*. It has a diagnostic medical code. The depression, if untreated, can result in suicide. It is a legitimate medical diagnosis and should be treated. This is obvious to healthcare providers who regularly treat these patients. At this time in the United States, children and adolescents are being treated with puberty blockers and hormones, but few under the age of 18 have undergone surgery. Multiple states are attempting to outlaw or limit the use of puberty-blocking drugs. The outlawing of surgery under the age of 18 may be prudent.

9

Arguments for and against Trans/DSD Athletes

There are many pro and con arguments for allowing trans athletes to compete. Most of the points are intuitive. Some are medically based. Many are speculative. The majority of arguments has become political/social. The main issue is athletes who identity as female and went through a male puberty and/or have an elevated testosterone level.

Pro Medical Argument

The main argument in favor of trans athletes is that testosterone does not make a difference. The basis of this is outdated studies that compared 100 elite athletes, both male and female, from different sports. It was found that somewhere between 5% and 15% of female athletes had testosterone levels that were in the lower male range, and 5–15% of male athletes' levels were in the upper female range. They decided from this that not all men have high testosterone levels and not all women have low testosterone. They concluded that testosterone does not really matter.

The problem with this is that they are looking at different unrelated sports such as golf and shooting, many of which are highly dependent on skill, and they did not include a lot of power and endurance sports, which are more dependent on testosterone. Intuitively, it does not make any sense that testosterone does not matter. It is important to have scientific studies because many things that seem obvious are more complex when studied scientifically. Quality studies on testosterone are lacking at this time.

Con Medical Argument

The con medical argument follows this logic: testosterone causes muscular development. It causes the development of strong bones and tendons as well as more cardiac and pulmonary capacity. This results in more aggressive behavior and neuromuscular wiring that leads to success in sports. It increases hemoglobin and red blood cells, thus oxygen-carrying capacity in endurance. Men beat women in most power and endurance sports. The presence of a Y chromosome, intrauterine testosterone, mini puberty, and adolescent puberty, along with a persistent testosterone level, result in an advantage to trans females that cannot be contested by a cis female. When a cis male has transitioned to a trans female, the residual effects of testosterone will never revert to a level comparable with a cis female. Some of the advantages of testosterone are permanent.

There may be individual outliers—cis female athletes who outperform trans males—but these are exceptions. There is not a large number of studies on this subject, but it makes intuitive sense. There are some sports that are not highly dependent on testosterone but rely on skill. This is why each sport needs to be considered on an individual basis. Many of these arguments ignore the DSD athlete, who is often not as straightforward a case as a trans athlete.

Pro Social Argument

Individuals who take a social, political, psychological, and/or human rights view believe that every child and adult has a right to participate in sports. Individuals with gender dysphoria have the right to change their sex to the sex that they feel most comfortable as. Gender identity can be fluid. Sports communities need to be cognizant of these facts. There are countries that prosecute and kill athletes for sexual orientation and gender identity. We need to remember this. Trans children have a right to participate in sports. Proponents often use the word *inclusive*.

Con Social Argument

The opposing social argument is that you are born a male or female, one or the other, and you cannot change your gender just because you feel you are in the wrong body. Proponents of this argument believe it is always unfair to have males competing against females. Not only is it unfair, but there is a chance of the trans female hurting the cis female. The trans males may also be injured by the cis males.

Arguments include the trans females taking away medals, scholarships, titles, team positions, and records from cis females. It is just plain unfair. These arguments are often based on emotion but very little scientific information.

Real Concerns

By now, it should be apparent that I believe in gender dysphoria as a medical entity and the right to transition gender when appropriately screened and supervised by medical individuals. I also believe it is something that begins in early childhood or in utero, whether the person acknowledges it or not. Surgery should be performed only on an adult unless it involves a DSD. Use of puberty-blocking drugs and hormones is generally safe and should be permitted in adolescents. Unlike surgery, the effects are theoretically reversible and not permanent. The subject of gender dysphoria, while not new to medicine, is only coming into acceptance now. What if their thoughts were to change on a subject with the accumulation of more data? In other words, what if the medical community is getting it wrong?

There have been situations in medicine where social or political thought and the government have influenced policy and changed the way medicine is practiced. It is worth presenting an example. Up until the 1990s, physicians used very few opioids or narcotics because of the addiction potential. Then the large drug companies started marketing an expensive form of a narcotic to physicians. They were so convincing that the medical community agreed and labeled pain as the "fifth vital sign." The way they represented pain was with a smiley face. Medicare believed the sales pitch and started to penalize physicians if they did not prescribe enough narcotics. The drug companies targeted less medically sophisticated medical environments. The results were disastrous, and it is the cause of the narcotics crisis that we are experiencing today. Are we making the same mistake with gender dysphoria? It is important to listen to critics of gender-confirmation surgery and not tune them out because they have different views from organized medicine.

We know that trans people have more depression and associated psychiatric issues. Is this because gender dysphoria is not addressed, or is it the other way around? Ideally, all trans patients should have counseling pre- and post-transition for a minimal amount of time. This is available through established programs. The duration of counseling is not universally agreed on. This should be prior to any drug administration and continue before and after any surgery. Since someone can transition privately, in this or another country, or even buy puberty-blocking drugs on the black market, it is impossible to regulate.

With a psychiatric evaluation, it might be discovered that gender-dysphoria patients have some other primary issue going on, with gender dysphoria being a secondary issue. This is a real concern with children and adolescents and also with certain groups, including autistic people, and those believed to have a primary diagnosis of depression.

Are people with gender dysphoria simply homosexuals? We discussed that in the section on orientation, and that does not appear to be the case. They are unrelated. Is the attraction to the appearance and dress of the opposite sex just a fetish? This was discussed in the "Crossdressers and Drag Queens" section in chapter 5 and is not the same issue.

Those in medicine must ask these questions and keep searching for the answers. Gender-confirmation surgery performed on a poorly selected subject is mutilation and battery. The same goes for children or adolescents below the age of consent, whatever that is determined to be. The ability of parents to consent for minors is still unclear. The role of puberty-blocking drugs should be embraced because they offer a generally safe and potentially reversible way of appropriate transition without a complete commitment until a certain period of time has passed and the person has reached a certain age.

10

Safe, Fair, and Inclusive Policies

It is important to remember that every country has different rules and uses different language. This can make it difficult to understand other countries' sports policies. Two phrases that come up commonly are *gender control,* which refers to assigning a person to the appropriate gender group, and *medical commission,* which refers to medical people making decisions. Both these terms are a little unusual in the United States.

In the United States, there are federal and state laws that affect trans/DSD athletes. The laws can be contradictory, and it is often unclear who has jurisdiction.

In the sports world, the IOC makes recommendations to the individual country's Olympic committees. In addition, each sport has an international and national governing body. The IOC has recommended that each sport establish its own policy recognizing that all sports are different. The recommendation of a medical commission to evaluate each athlete individually has not universally occurred yet, though it has in some countries. There are other organizations such as the National Collegiate Athletic Association (NCAA) and High School Sports Association that may also have jurisdiction. The rules are often contradictory, and this creates much confusion.

It is important to remember that in some situations, there are just as many trans male athletes as trans female. Trans male athletes do not receive much publicity because of the partly false belief that they do not win. There have been gifted cis female athletes who transition to trans male athletes to play up against a much more competitive field with little hope of winning. This has occurred in NCAA sports and is used as an argument in favor of trans athletes. It is clear that the desire to correct one's gender presentation outweighs the desire to win an athletic event.

Title IX is the 1975 US federal law giving female athletes an equal opportunity in sports and education in institutions that receive federal funds. This includes elementary schools, high schools, colleges, and universities. It allows such things as girls being able to play on boys' teams when there are no girls' teams available. It has also allowed girls to play with boys in situations where the girls' team is not competitive. It mandates equal opportunity and scholarships for girls.

This was originally interpreted by trans athletes' proponents to mean that trans girls cannot be discriminated against in sports. In 2020, there was a bill known as the Protection of Women in Sports Act, which sought to ban all the trans women and trans girls from school athletic programs. It would only recognize gender if there was associated birth-sex and biological congruency. There are still trans-athlete activists who want to have Title IX changed to include gender identity and sexual orientation. In 2023, the US Education Department stated that school policy may not categorically ban trans athletes, but in some instances, it may limit their participation. In this situation, they would still be compliant with Title IX. On the state level in the United States, at the time this book is being written, there are over 20 states that ban trans athletes and over 40 bills pending in state legislatures.

World Athletics, which is the international body of track and field, instituted a new policy in 2023. Trans women who have gone through a cis male puberty would be banned from female world-ranking competitions. This would essentially be all international competitions. It also set the testosterone level for DSD athletes at 2.5 nmol/L. This is particularly important because there are currently over a dozen world-class track and field athletes with a DSD. With the new rules, all would require six months' reduction in testosterone to a specific level in order to compete.

Safe, fair, and inclusive has become the motto for trans/DSD athletes. While it would be ideal to come up with a policy that meets all three requirements, it is unlikely to happen in all sports. Safety is an issue in contact sports, while fairness is an issue in most testosterone-dependent sports. Safe and fair go hand in hand but often are inconsistent with inclusiveness. People who advocate for inclusiveness often have a social agenda and ignore the medical facts. To satisfy all three requirements would necessitate every sport to be considered separately and every athlete individually. There definitely will be situations where athletes are left out.

In 2022, NCAA swimming adopted a new transgender rule, which it termed as a "gender inclusion policy." It allows trans female athletes who meet the testosterone requirements of one year suppression to compete. This ruling follows World Aquatics rulings that trans female athletes are excluded from international competition. World Aquatics is the governing body of water sports in the world. It has started an open category, although no one has yet registered.

In the spring of 2021, Caitlyn Jenner, Olympic gold medalist and noted trans woman, spoke out against trans women competing with cis women. The positive outcome of all these rules is that the sports world is considering each sport differently. It is also distinguishing between trans and DSD athletes. They are realizing the importance of mini puberty and testosterone levels and viewing issues as more of a medical problem and not just a social situation.

World Athletics Policy

World Athletics, the international sports organization of track and field, has followed the IOC recommendations and written a trans/DSD athletic policy. Many organizations have started to make policies, but they have been mostly sociopolitical and lacking medical guidance. The policies have been more trans-athlete oriented and less DSD-athlete specific. World Athletics has written a policy that addresses both, is medically based, and offers recommendations regarding whether or not an athlete is qualified to compete. This policy will certainly be revised and improved in the future, but at this time, in my opinion, it is the best policy to date.

Track and field events are very athletically dependent, and it is believed that testosterone plays an important role in performance. There have been multiple studies on testosterone in track and field. In the new policy, trans females who went through cis male puberty are currently excluded from international competition. DSD athletes are evaluated by the type of DSD they have as well as their individual medical findings, particularly their testosterone level. Many of these DSD athletes are able to compete if their testosterone is below 2.5 nmol/L for six months prior to the competition. While it is possible to find fault in the policy, it is certainly a step in the right direction.

World Aquatics and other organizations such as the NCAA are starting to develop significant policies that contain points similar to the World Athletics policy. At this point, the policies are still a little complex and difficult to understand.

Compromise Policies

Compromise policies are policies generated by arbitration and compromise. They tend to be early policies and are high on sociopolitical ideas and lack scientific medical data. Suggested policies have included such concepts as having an additional open division that trans and DSD athletes can compete in. Others have suggested letting trans/DSD athletes play in the regular pool but not allowing medals, titles, scholarships, or records. All these policies seem reasonable in theory, but they may not be practical. Opponents of compromise policies have described them as "cutting the baby in half."

Confusing Policy

Recently USA Boxing came out with a trans policy that is inconsistent with other sports organizations. The policy states that minor athletes must compete in birth-assigned gender groups. It states that trans women may compete with cis women if they have undergone gender reassignment surgery (details omitted). They will also need to maintain a testosterone level bellow 5 nmol/L for four years with quarterly blood monitoring.

The exclusion of minor-age athletes is unusual since most sports rely on a large pool of child athletes to develop their adult champions. It is a known fact that the majority of gender-identity issues start in childhood.

The requirement of gender reassignment surgery is archaic and has not been part of any trans policy in over 20 years. This suggests the lack of clear understanding between gender identity and biologic sex.

If a cis male were to have gender reassignment surgery, it would include castration, making the testosterone level less than 2.5 nmol/L. In this case, the athlete would only require routine drug testing, not quarterly testosterone levels. This four-year period of low testosterone is a more reasonable direction, understanding that a full hormone transition can take as long as six years. The testosterone level of below 5 nmol/L is not consistent with other policies.

What makes this policy confusing is that it is different than most current sports organization policies. It ignores the effects of testosterone during puberty, which is at the center of trans athlete controversy. Boxing is a combat sport, and combat sports are thought to be the most dangerous for trans athletes.

11

Author's Proposed Policies

In a prior publication, I outlined the scheme for trans and DSD athletes to participate in competitive sports. This earlier plan was for the sport of judo. Judo is a vigorous power, strength, and contact sport. It is a combat sport. This plan was early in the discussion of trans athletes, and issues like mini puberty, Y chromosomes, and neurological effects of testosterone were not mentioned very much in the literature. This was okay because most of the concern is male puberty and testosterone levels.

While the proposed plan for judo served as a good introduction, it became clear that each sport would have to establish its own plan. What applies to judo, a combat sport, may not apply to a sport like shooting or curling. This is not to detract from or minimize the physical skill needed for those sports. Some sports are more dependent on skill than strength and power. In these sports, testosterone may not be as major a factor, but it is still relevant.

With the multitude of DSDs in addition to trans athletes in a great variety of sports, it will likely be necessary to establish a medical commission to evaluate each individual athlete. It is possible that some sports will have limited competitive participation, although it is hoped that recreational sports will remain open to all. All children and adults have a need and a right to participate in physical activity as long as it is safe and fair. This is the inclusivity that must be part of any policy.

In some sports, when a scholarship, record, title, or medal is at stake, it may not be fair. These discussions need to be based on medical knowledge and not emotions. Some have suggested having open, trans, and nonelite divisions to solve the problem. Many of these compromise solutions are weak. In time, a medical and scientific policy will evolve. Whatever it is, it must be a balance between safety and fairness and not just inclusivity.

Trans Athletes

Prepubertal Athletes: This refers to child athletes. Prepubertal trans boys and girls can play in either the male or female division. In many sports, these groups are mixed. In most of the world, boys and girls play sports in a mixed-sex group until about 10 years of age, when cis girls start puberty and have an advantage over boys. Girls usually start puberty a year or two before boys.

Trans Male Athletes: In this group, it does not matter if the transition was done pre- or postpuberty, although, theoretically, a prepubertal transition would more closely align with a cis boy. This is because the effects of estrogen would be blocked, and with the effects of testosterone, the child would more closely resemble a cis boy. If a trans boy did a postpubertal transition, there should still be a strong effect of the testosterone, but female secondary sex characteristics such as breasts would have to be dealt with.

These athletes would have to have declared their gender identity and have been on testosterone replacement for an agreed-on amount of time. Because these athletes will have had a transition with testosterone, many people might count this as a "male puberty." It is recommended that if they reconsidered and wanted to go back to a female identity, they should have an extended period of no play, probably about four years. Some national and international associations might permanently bar this athlete from competition as a cis female.

These athletes, like all, would need a TUE for each drug taken to be in compliance with WADA. The main concern with these athletes, particularly in contact sports like judo, is the risk of hurting themselves. It is possible that some contact or combat sports would exclude most postpuberty trans male athletes. The rules must be designed to prevent injury and provide safety to the athlete, particularly children, regardless of the social point of view.

Prepubertal Transition Trans Female Athletes: Athletes who transition prepubertally to female, without exposure to testosterone, are generally accepted to be a special situation. The major effects of testosterone are strongest in the adolescent male. Boys who have avoided adolescent puberty despite Y chromosomes, intrauterine hormones, and mini puberty are generally very close to cis females. Most sports organizations, including World Athletics, will accept these trans female athletes. These children might never have had elevated testosterone and would have been treated with Lupron and estrogen replacement at puberty.

Postpubertal Transition Trans Female Athletes: This is one of the main obstacles in trans athletics. These athletes have gone through adolescent puberty with testosterone, and even though they may have transitioned for two or more years (as most organizations require), the effects of the testosterone are generally irreversible. Many sports organizations are moving to banning these athletes from competitions. This is a sport-by-sport decision. If allowed to play, these athletes would have to be below an acceptable level for an accepted period of time. People have suggested a cis female level for a two-year period. Most sports might choose to ban these athletes.

DSD Athletes

What makes a DSD athlete different is that they were born with a medical issue, unlike the trans athlete, who has a gender dysphoria issue.

Complete Androgen Insensitivity Syndrome: This is a genotypic XY male who lacks testosterone receptors. The testosterone has no effect. The Y chromosome is present, but its effect and the absence of testosterone function are thought to be minimal, if any. These individuals phenotypically appear to be female. They usually are statistically taller than cis females but not enough to confer any athletic advantage. In theory, they should have an elevated testosterone level, but in practice, levels are variable. The effect of testosterone on hemoglobin and hematocrit development is unknown but thought to be minimal if present.

These individuals can be treated as females and play as that gender without any concern about an advantage. It is important that they are certified as CAIS and not PAIS, which is discussed in the next section. Some sports organizations may include all DSDs together and require a testosterone level of 2.5 nmol/L for a certain period of time. This is not necessary with this DSD. This is actually one of the more straightforward DSDs to deal with. There is no adolescent puberty here.

Partial Androgen Insensitivity Syndrome: The problem with this DSD is that it occurs in many different forms in varying degrees of androgen insensitivity. Some affected individuals are very close to female phenotype and some closer to male. When they phenotypically resemble males and identify as a male, there is no problem. If they identify as a female, some believe it is better for them to be treated as trans individuals. This needs to be determined on a case-by-case basis.

Because people with PAIS have partial androgen function, they fall into a diagnosis of female gender identity DSD athletes with elevated testosterone. Some people would want to treat them as trans females and some as DSD athletes. This is why individual sports organizations require a medical commission with consideration of each athlete as an individual. Right now, most organizations consider PAIS a DSD. The reason this is considered a DSD and not as trans female is because there is a naturally occurring medical condition and not pure gender dysphoria.

Mild Androgen Insensitivity Syndrome: Individuals with MAIS are phenotypically male, and most will have a cis male gender identity, but they can also be trans female. If they have a cis male identity, they are treated as males. If they are trans females, they are best treated as part of a trans female group and not a DSD group. The issue here is whether or not they have experienced male adolescent puberty. This is a diagnosis that is very diverse and may require individual medical consultation. The patients often are seen in the urologist's office with nonspecific diagnosis, erectile issues, and minor genitourinary anomalies.

Adrenal Cortical Hyperplasia (Adrenal Genital Syndrome) in Males XY: This discussion is restricted to 21-hydroxylase deficiency, which makes it more than 95% ACH. The other enzyme deficiencies that occur in ACH are rare and need to be evaluated on an individual basis, but 21-hydroxylase deficiency is the most common DSD in the world and the most common XX DSD.

XY males with ACH may require medication as a child and may or may not need to remain on it as an adult. In theory, they can have a high testosterone level because they lack an adrenal enzyme. This causes an increased production of the testosterone predecessors, which results in increased testosterone and other adrenal androgens.

In reality, they usually have a normal testosterone range. Male athletes with ACH have been known to occasionally fail a drug test for testosterone or other androgens. If they require any other medications such as a cortisone or mineral corticoids, they are required to have the appropriate TUE. Most males with ACH encountered it at infancy and not at adulthood. Most compete in sports as a male with no issues.

Adrenal Cortical Hyperplasia (Adrenal Genital Syndrome) in Females XX: ACH in females is sometimes an issue in sports. These females have a deficiency of 21-hydroxylase and produce excess levels of androgens and testosterone. The overproduction is necessary for their survival. The androgens can result in an increased size of the clitoris, and there is confusion as to the child's phenotypic sex. They can appear masculine or at least ambiguous at birth. They usually require cortisone and mineral corticoids as an infant and perhaps as an adult. They may require surgical procedures such as clitoral reduction (making the clitoris smaller so it does not look like a penis), which is performed as an infant. For this reason, gender identity issues are thought to be below 30%. These patients are often not gender dysphoric enough to want to transition to a male. They just tend to be more masculine women.

The problems are with congenitally high testosterone and other androgens in a female gender identity. Since it is a DSD in an XX female, most sports organizations require testosterone reduction to 2.5 nmol/L. There is no concern for male puberty here. Most of these athletes, as adults, have normal testosterone for a female but may require medications. A TUE would, of course, be necessary. These athletes usually compete as women with no problems.

5-Alpha Reductase Deficiency: This was once thought to be a rare diagnosis, but this syndrome is becoming more and more common in athletes. It has been suggested that 5-ARD confers an advantage to an athlete who identifies as female gender. 5-ARD is a DSD with an XY (male genotype) and usually a female gender identity. If the individual is XX (female genotype), the lack of 5-ARD enzyme is insignificant since women do not have much testosterone. If the XY genotype 5-ARD identifies as a male, there is no issue, although, theoretically, they could have elevated testosterone. In reality, this does not happen.

When lacking an enzyme to convert testosterone to dihydroxy testosterone, its active form, this deficiency is often overcome at puberty because of high testosterone levels with subsequent masculinization of an XY phenotypic female. This has led some researchers to believe that these individuals undergo a natural cis male adolescent puberty and should be classified as a trans athlete and not a DSD athlete. Current rules classify them as a DSD athlete and call for regulation of their testosterone level to 2.5 nmol/L. Since they were classified as trans athletes who went through puberty, they would be ineligible to play in many sports organizations. Critics of trans athletes argue that they should not be allowed to compete in sports. Proponents argue that the puberty is not significant because the testosterone may not be fully functional; thus, they should be treated as any other DSD athlete. At this time, it is generally believed that they are DSD athletes and should have their testosterone at the appropriate level without regard to puberty.

Other DSDs: Other DSDs, of which at least 60 have been identified, would have to be evaluated on an individual basis. Many of the categories outlined in this section can serve as a guide to their evaluation. They would require an expert medical panel (medical commission) for each sports organization. Each athlete would need to be evaluated, usually by medical records from their treating physician, before a discussion could be started. There would be a number of athletes who would not fit into any of the above criteria, and if no decision could be made on their eligibility, they might need to be excluded from competition. Medicine is an art as well as a science, and it does not always have an exact answer. It would be assumed that the sports community would listen to the decision of the medical commission. A sample athlete evaluation form is included below.

Sample Medical Evaluation Form for DSD/Trans Athletes

Name:

Age:

Height:

Weight:

Sex Assigned at Birth:

Genotype / Karyotype:

Phenotype / Genital Appearance:

Gender Identity:

Gender Presentation:

Existing DSD Diagnosis:

Natural T Level and Electrolytes:

Current Medications:

Recent T Level (within Three Months):

Other Medical Diagnoses:

Depression / Psych Screening:

Sports / Level of Play:

Substance Abuse:

Understanding of Issues and Process:

Declaration of Gender and Duration:

Desire to Transition:

Desire to Play as a DSD/Trans Athlete:

Parent Understanding:

Parent Support:

12

Caster Semenya– A Case Study

Caster Semenya is a South African middle-distance runner and 2016 Olympic gold medalist. She first came to attention when she greatly improved her time in the 800 meters event. She actually took eight seconds off her prior best performance, which brought her under the scrutiny of the local sports association. She was also very muscular, and this created some concerns. Nobody considered the possibility that she was just training very hard and was just a naturally, genetically gifted athlete. There were other athletes who fit into this category, and the extra scrutiny she was put under was discriminatory.

She has become the most famous DSD athlete in the world. Most of the information available has been leaked by the media. She has been a victim of multiple contradictory court rulings, and the situation is quite confusing. Her story can serve as an illustration of the issues.

In reviewing the literature online, it is unclear which DSD Caster Semenya has. She actually is reported to have three or four different disorders. Further, it is actually no one's business other than hers, her physician's, and any sports organization she releases her medical records to. Someone's medical records are private and confidential and should not be leaked to the media. Since we are not her physicians and not treating her, we did not have her permission to discuss her medical condition. What condition she has is therefore irrelevant. This a recurrent issue in the world of sports with issues of gender identity and DSDs. It is time for the athletic community, particularly sports organizations, to respect the athlete and deal with these matters appropriately, with confidentiality and through a sports-specific medical commission. She has been cited as a DSD athlete in the past because of her great athletic success. She is one of over a dozen DSD athletes in organized sports with similar problems. DSD athletes are not uncommon in female track and field.

It is again important to stress that we do not know her medical history or current medical condition. In May 2020, the Board of Arbitration of Sports (BAS) ruled that Caster Semenya cannot compete in international track because of a congenitally high testosterone level. The court ruled that women who have high testosterone levels are at an unfair advantage in certain track and field events. Prior to this, they had restricted her from competing in certain events but not others. The court acknowledged that this was a prejudicial ruling because it was due to a naturally occurring medical condition but that the rule was necessary for fairness toward the other athletes.

In 2021, BAS barred her from competing in the 400-meter, 800-meter, 1,500-meter, and one-mile events. This was based on a 2017 paper in the *British Journal of Sports Medi-*

cine concluding that these events are most testosterone-dependent. Most authorities believed the article to be flawed at the time it was published. World Athletics (the governing body for track and field) subsequently stated a testosterone level of 5 nmol/L for DSD athletes in these events and most recently lowered it to 2.5 nmol/L for all DSD athletes.

Caster Semenya subsequently competed in the 5,000-meter event, which is longer than a mile, prior to the 2020 Olympics. She did well but was not able to qualify for the Olympic Games. Critics of trans/DSD athletes have attributed this to the longer distance being less testosterone-dependent. Others argue that all events are as likely to be dependent as not. In theory, testosterone should increase hemoglobin in oxygen-carrying capacity, which would help longer-distance runners. It is more likely that some people are just better in some events than others or that she was already too old to pick up a new event and be competitive.

There was talk in 2020 that Caster Semenya was going to switch to football (soccer), although this has not happened to date. Apparently, she would not be under the same scrutiny with football rules. Currently, she is coaching and working on her distance running. Being 30 years old, she is likely too old to start her career as a sprinter. Sprinting can be more stressful on the tendons and muscles as one ages. She has also become an author, writing an autobiography, which was published in November 2023.

In the summer of 2021, the *British Journal of Sport Medicine* corrected the article on testosterone in track events. Currently, World Athletics sets DSD athletes' testosterone level at 2.5 nmol/L and prohibits all trans females who went through a male puberty from competition. DSD athletes continue to argue that their testosterone is naturally occurring and it would be a violation of their human rights to have to change it. Some DSD athletes refuse to take medication to lower their testosterone. This is why Caster Semenya initially switched to distance events. With today's rules, she would be ineligible for all events unless she lowered her testosterone.

There have been some concerns regarding race issues with Caster Semenya. This has been suggested because she is a person of color. More recently, she has been used as an illustration of the lack of medical care available to those who are impoverished worldwide. If she had come from a more affluent society, she may have had her DSD treated as a child and not had any issues as an adult. The last concern involving race and DSDs is a possible increased frequency in certain racial groups. Since DSDs are genetic traits that tend to cluster in geographically isolated groups, evidence suggests an ethnic component to most DSDs but not a racial predilection. DSD seems to occur in diverse racial populations.

Confidentiality

As stated above, medical records are private and confidential and, at least in the United States, protected by state and federal law. There have been recent concerns about trans athletes competing in sports without disclosing their status. At this point, there are no laws requiring a person to disclose their status. It is simply a matter of honesty and ethics. If the consent form for the sporting event asks one's gender status, it might be possible to obtain that information as a prerequisite to competing in the event.

When the human immunodeficiency virus (HIV) first became widespread, there were laws prohibiting positive individuals from engaging in contact sports. When it was realized that it had a low transmissibility, these laws were replaced by anti-discriminatory laws that made it illegal to stop someone from participating in a sport because of their HIV status. Almost all government forms ask questions about gender identity. This is likely to occur with sports entry forms and consent in the near future.

Conclusion

This is a challenging subject, but it can be summarized in this conclusion. There are two groups to consider, trans athletes and DSD athletes. The medical community, particularly in the United States and the Western world, accepts gender dysphoria and trans people as a medical reality. People with DSDs have always been a medical reality. The difference here should not be in whether to recognize and accept these two groups but in understanding how they fit into sports.

The main debate revolves around testosterone and cis male adolescent puberty. There is also a concern over DSD athletes who identify with the female gender with an elevated testosterone level regardless of their genotype. These DSD athletes are less scrutinized because they are accepted as a medical malady.

Each sport is different and must individually determine the role that testosterone plays in the sport and if it is appropriate to have trans/DSD athletes playing. The motto "safe and fair" needs to be followed, and only then can inclusiveness be considered. Once a sport is established, guidelines and individual medical commissions will likely be necessary to evaluate each trans and DSD athlete—particularly the latter—on an individual basis. An athlete who is eligible in one sport may not be eligible in another.

At the time of publication, there is a clear trend to prohibit trans female athletes who went through male puberty and to require low testosterone levels in DSD athletes for a certain period of time prior to competition. As we have seen, our knowledge is constantly being redefined, and the rules that govern trans/DSD athletes are changing. This book will quickly become out of date, which is a good thing, because its purpose is to stimulate discussion and not serve as an authoritative text.

Bibliography

American Psychiatric Association, *Diagnostic and Statistical Manual of Mental Disorders, Fifth Edition* (DSM-5-TR). Washington, DC: American Psychiatric Publishing Inc., 2023.

Bermon, Stephane, Pierre-Yves Garnier. "Serum Androgen Levels and Their Relationship to Performance in Track and Field: Mass Spectrometry from 2,127 Observations in Male and Female Elite Athletes." *British Journal of Sports Medicine* (September 2017): j51:1309-14 Volume 51, Issue 17.

Bermon, Stephane, Pierre-Yves Garnier, et al. *British Journal of Sports Medicine* correction electronic page (September 2021): Volume 51, Issue 17.

Catanese, Anthony J. *The Medical Care of the Judoka.* Expanded edition. Arizona: Wheatmark, 2022.

Catanese, Anthony J. *The Medical Care of the Judoka.* Arizona: Wheatmark, 2012.

"International Judo Federation Sports and Organization

Rules" (update 2022-2024): published online Documents www.IJF.org.

International Olympic Committee (IOC) Statement on Sex Change Operations: online www.olympics.com/ioc.

Judo Canada. "Policy on Transgender Athletics" (August 7, 2017): online www.judocanada.org.

Medicine and Science in Sports and Exercise (2010–2023). Issues 1–12, Volumes 42–55.

National Collegiate Athletic Association. "Transgender Student-Athlete Participation Policy" (January 2022, updated April 2023): online www.ncaa.org/transgender.

Roger I. Dmochowski, Luis R. Kavoussi, Craig A. Peters, and Alan J. Wein. *Campbell-Walsh-Wein Urology, Twelfth Edition Review*. Philadephia, St Louis, New York: Elsevier, 2022.

Title IX, Education Amendments Act of 1972, 20 U.S.C.

USA Judo Medical Committee. Trans Athlete Policy Discussion. Committee meetings 2023-2024.

USJF Medical Committee. Trans Athlete Policy Discussion. Committee meetings 2023.

World Aquatics Trans Policy (2023): online www.worldaquatics.com.

World Athletics Trans/DSD Policy (March 2023): online www.worldathletics.org.

About the Author

Anthony J. Catanese, MD, is a board-certified urologist who has been practicing medicine for over 40 years. He completed his residency at New York University/Bellevue. In addition to adult and pediatric urology, he is also trained in emergency medicine and sports medicine. He is a Fellow of the American College and the International College of Surgeons as well as a member of the American College of Sports Medicine.

Dr. Catanese is a judo player with 60 years' experience and holds the rank of sixth-degree black belt. He has served as the USA Judo Team physician at five world championships. Having served on the International Judo Federation Medical Commission and the TUE subcommittee, he is well versed in the organization of sports on an international level. In the United States, he has worked with the US Judo Federation and USA Judo to develop a trans/DSD policy for athletes. In his practice, he regularly treats trans/DSD athletes.

Early in his career, he worked in a large obstetrical hospital, which enabled him to regularly see newborns with DSD. As part of the team of healthcare practitioners, he participated in the diagnosis and treatment of DSD children. Later in his career, he was a member of a large urologic practice that performed gender-confirmation surgery.

As a sports medicine and US sports team physician, he has been involved with WADA and other world organizations in the abuse of testosterone.

One of Dr. Catanese's greatest skills as a physician has been his ability to explain difficult topics. This book's purpose is to introduce information on a difficult subject to the sports community so that informed, intelligent, and non-emotional discussions can be had.

www.ingramcontent.com/pod-product-compliance
Lightning Source LLC
Chambersburg PA
CBHW072004150726
47999CB00002B/510